AMERICAN PLAGUES

Lessons from Our Battles
with Disease

D1155241

NOTICE

AMERICAN PLAGUES

Lessons from Our Battles with Disease

STEPHEN H. GEHLBACH, MD, MPH
University of Massachusetts
Amherst, Massachusetts

McGraw-Hill
Medical Publishing Division

New York   Chicago   San Francisco   Lisbon   London   Madrid
Mexico City   Milan   New Delhi   San Juan   Seoul
Singapore   Sydney   Toronto

Copyright © 2005 by The McGraw-Hill Companies, Inc. All rights reserved. Printed in the United States of America. Except as permitted under the United States Copyright Act of 1976, no part of this publication may be reproduced or distributed in any form or by any means, or stored in a data base or retrieval system, without prior written permission of the publisher.

1 2 3 4 5 6 7 8 9 0   DOC/DOC   0 9 8 7 6 5 4

ISBN 0-07-143790-8

This book was set in Palatino by International Typesetting and Composition.
The editors were Isabel Nogueira and Christie Naglieri.
The production supervisor was Catherine Saggese.
The cover designer was Aimee Nordin.
The index was prepared by Robert P. Swanson.
RR Donnelley was the printer and binder.

This book is printed on acid-free paper.

Library of Congress Cataloging-in-Publication Data

Stephen H. Gehlbach.
    American plagues: lessons from our battles with disease/edited by Stephen H. Gehlbach.—1st ed.
      p.;   cm.
    Includes bibliographical references and index.
    ISBN # 0-07-143790-8 (softcover)
1. Epidemics—United States—History.   2. Epidemiology. I. Gehlbach, Stephen H.
[DNLM: 1. Disease Outbreaks—history—United States.   2. Communicable Disease Control—history—United States.   3. Epidemiology—History—United States. WA 11 AA1 A512 2004]
    RA650.5. A57 2004
    614.4'0973—dc22   2004049971

CONTENTS

My first encounter with epidemiology came in a spare, window-less room in the headquarters of Atlanta's Centers for Disease Control and Prevention. Together with some 40 other new recruits to the Epidemic Intelligence Service, I was immersed in a crash course to learn the techniques of this critical science. Over several weeks we were expected to master sufficient skills to help departments throughout the country protect the public's health. We were learning to become medical detectives, to solve the riddles of the causes of unexpected clusters of disease.

—A church supper has just been spoiled by an outbreak of food poisoning. Dozens are afflicted with severe gastrointestinal distress. Does the pattern of illness point to a source among the various foods consumed? How do you decide which one?

—A small Michigan community reports a sudden rise in cases of hepatitis. Is the apparent link to a local doughnut shop just a coincidence?

It was a fascinating challenge. And that one brief summer course was just the beginning. It turned out that the principles required to find the cause of food-poisoning could be applied to the complexities of cancer and heart disease. The common reasoning tools and thought processes could help to explain a host of diseases and how one might prevent them. The detective game had wide application and yielded valuable results.

In the years since then I've tried to make epidemiology contagious: pass it on to medical and public health students who need to understand how diseases operate in populations and how best to control them. Its principles—the study of illness in human groups and the techniques devised to carry out the work—form the basis for much of what we know about our health: how diseases come about, how they are "caught" and spread, and how we can evaluate their prevention and cure.

This book is intended for all those who wish to know such things. Students of public health as well as those in professional health science careers should find that it supplies a grounding in the principles of epidemiologic thought. For students in the early parts of their careers—in public health, medicine, nursing, or allied health fields—the concepts found in any introductory text of epidemiology are here. Mid-career professionals should find that the book provides an opportunity to re-examine ideas encountered in their past or the chance to explore a new domain.

The book is also aimed at a broader audience—all those who have an interest in our collective struggles with disease. General readers should find help in making sense of health reports that cascade down upon us from the print and broadcast media. The bulk of this news is based on medical and public health research, and these chapters should make it more intelligible. Included for this group is some essential background information: basic descriptions of how diseases operate, the ways in which hostile agents inflict their damage, the symptoms they produce, and rudiments of the complex subject of immune response.

The principles elucidated here all have a context. They emerge from narratives of our struggles with the nation's epidemics—plagues past and present. The stories span three centuries beginning with smallpox and continuing through our ongoing confrontations with AIDS and SARS. Protagonists include doctors and clergy, writers and newsmen, public health institutions, and even a town. The stories are quite human—filled with ambition and accomplishment, jealousy and disappointment, public spirit and self-interest, egotism and modesty, self-sacrifice and self-delusion. Some episodes lead to vital discoveries, new ways of understanding and improving human health. Others proved unproductive. But all held the prospect of finding something new. I hope these chapters will help readers make their own discoveries.

This book owes much to the support of others. Shauna Seliy and Janet Kellogg gave research and manuscript assistance. Kristin Meadows, Kyna Hamill, Anne Sauer, and Esta Schindler helped locate illustrations. Isabel Nogueira offered sustaining encouragement. Special appreciation goes to Kit Fairchild, Hilary Conklin, and Hunter Gehlbach for critiques and technical aid. And most of all I thank my wife Carol. She knows what I mean.

Stephen H. Gehlbach, MD, MPH

CHAPTER 1

Gunpowder and Calomel: Benjamin Rush and the Malignant Yellow Fever

It was well after ten o'clock and the mid-September evening in 1793 was turning unusually cool. Benjamin Rush picked up his pen to write. "My dear, Julia," Rush began, to his wife who, though only 30 miles distant in New Jersey, seemed a world away. The chill in the air had refreshed him slightly, but he was bone weary. Weeks of frantic work and little sleep had taken their toll. He had been visiting as many as 100 patients each day in every part of the city. Patients had crowded outside his home and he had even had to write prescriptions seated at his supper table. In the past few days he, himself, had fallen ill and had been forced to curtail practice. But the anguish of not tending to his patients had overridden his own discomforts. People were desperate for his assistance. "For some days before my confinement," he wrote to Julia, "I refused from 50 to 60 patients a day. This was a most painful task. Many of them left me in tears. One man, a sailor, offered me 20 pounds to visit his wife, but I declined it. In riding through town I was often stopped by half a dozen people, all imploring me to visit a wife, a husband, a brother, or a child. Judge how I must have felt in tearing myself from them, for I could only visit a certain number and by undertaking more than I could attend, some I knew would die from neglect" (1, pp. 668–669).

That morning he had resumed his rounds. "I have this day visited one family in the neighborhood on foot, and four at a distance in a carriage, and feel so well after it that tomorrow I expect to visit a dozen or twenty" (1, pp. 668–669). It was a note of hope in an otherwise unhappy situation. The scenes that Rush had been encountering earlier in the day and in the preceding weeks offered little comfort. Nothing was normal. As he had passed the covered market between Front Street and Second Street, he found it almost deserted. Stalls customarily overflowing with produce from the fertile New Jersey farms across the river were largely deserted—the farmers forgoing profits in favor of safety. There were almost no livestock for sale and butchers had only scraps remaining. The few vendors who had stayed guarded their posts warily. Some clutched handkerchiefs in their hands, which they sprinkled periodically with vinegar. These they brought quickly to their noses when customers approached. Other kept piles of garlic close at hand and chewed the cloves continually. Still others had small bags of camphor tied about their necks or laced upon their shoes.

Customers were also sparse. Those who were about, seemed hunted. They eyed each other suspiciously and avoided contact. Strangers gave especially wide berth to one another, but even among friends greetings were perfunctory. No handshakes or embraces were exchanged. People kept to the middle of the street as if fearing to come near the vendors or the homes that lined the street beyond the market. Few children were in evidence and those who could be seen were wrapped in amulets of garlic or camphor. Some had even taken up tobacco. Rush witnessed two small boys not more than 10 years old smoking "seegars" in front of Christ Church on Second Street.

Closer to the river the scene was stranger still. Water Street was almost deserted. Absent was the usual bustle of the busy port, the dock hands unloading cargos, the carts of sugar and molasses clattering over stones; the streets sat almost silent. The groaning wheels of mortuary carts were the only sounds of commerce. Fitful bursts of musket fire were also heard along the street; they came from no particular direction and had had no apparent purpose. At the corners of Race and Arch streets unattended bonfires still smoldered. Most of the homes, shops, taverns, and warehouses were shut. The scene reminded Rush of war.

Indeed, Philadelphia was a city under siege. But the enemy was not in view. The attack came not, as it had 15 years earlier, from British Redcoats, nor from their complicit Hessian mercenaries, nor from any human force. The enemy in the late summer of 1793 was disease—a malignant fever that was spreading rapidly and taking far more lives than any foreign army might. Only one month had passed since Rush had first recognized the danger, and already there had been 970 deaths, with more occurring every day.

August 19 was the date that Rush made his discovery. He had been called to assist Dr. Hodge and Dr. Foulke with Mrs. LeMaigre, the wife of a prosperous merchant who resided on Water Street. Her appearance alarmed him immediately. On entering the home he had seen her desperate condition, the raging fever, the rapid pulse, the yellowing eyes and skin. "She vomited constantly and complained of great heat and burning in her stomach," he wrote. As Rush discussed the situation with his colleagues, his alarm increased. Dr. Hodge had reported "that a fever of a most malignant kind had carried off four or five persons within the sight of Mrs. LeMaigre's door, and that one of them had died twelve hours after the attack of the disease" (2, p. 43). Rush himself had attended an unusual number of similar cases in the same neighborhood over the past week. Then doctor Foulke revealed more chilling news. At the end of July a ship from the West Indies had dumped a load of spoiled coffee on Mr. Ball's wharf only a short distance from the LeMaigre house. The decaying coffee had produced a penetrating, noxious odor that permeated the neighborhood. As Rush reflected on his recent cases, Mrs. Bradford and her sister Mrs. Leaming, young Mr. McNair and Mrs. Palmer's two sons, and Mr. Alston had all been in the neighborhood and had been exposed to the exhalations. These cases were not instances of the typical late summer fevers that frequented Philadelphia every year. They were too concentrated, too severe. As Rush assembled the facts before him he could reach only one conclusion, that Philadelphia was in the grip of an epidemic malignant fever—bilious yellow fever.

His was a bold revelation, one that would provoke argument from colleagues and high anxiety in the citizenry. But Rush was up to the challenge. At age 47, he was a man of some standing in Philadelphia. His signature was on the Declaration of Independence and he had served his nation bravely in the recent War for Independence. His medical training was excellent. After serving an apprenticeship with the highly respected Dr. Redman of Philadelphia, he did what many able and ambitious young American doctors did, he shipped himself across the Atlantic to polish his education. He studied for two years in Edinburgh, at the time the Mecca of medical thought in Europe. There he was heavily influenced by his mentor, Dr. Cullen, whose theories on the causes and classification of diseases were at the vanguard of medical opinion.

Rush was only 22 when he returned to Philadelphia, but the educational credentials he brought back positioned him among the medical elite in the new republic. He wasted little time in putting his training to use and was soon elected professor of chemistry at the College of Philadelphia. His private practice began more slowly. Rush was of a modest background. His father had been a gunsmith and, upon the father's death, Benjamin's mother had opened a small grocery store above Second Street near the market when Benjamin was 5 years old. The family lacked the social connections that would assure their son association with more affluent patients. Eager to try his trade regardless of the financial consequences, Rush attended the less well-to-do. He soon earned a reputation for the energy and dedication he brought to his practice. (See Figure 1-1.)

His position as a medical opinion leader had grown over the years. In 1787, he had been a founder of the first College of Physicians in Philadelphia and two years later became professor of practice at the college that was to become the University of Pennsylvania. He had written and lectured widely, and his opinion carried weight.

So when Rush placed a statement in the local paper that the malignant yellow fever was upon the town, people paid attention. Word spread rapidly and, as the number of cases of yellow fever grew, so did fear. People applied whatever measures were available to protect themselves. For many, the response was flight. Families with transportation and relatives outside of town gathered essential belongings and headed out. Throughout the last week of August and first weeks of September, the streets were cluttered with carriages and carts. Any conveyance that could transport people away from the danger was appropriated. Rush reported to his wife Julia, "Our neighborhood will be desolate in a day or two. Dr. White's, Mrs. Chew's and Mr. Louis' families are all on the wing" (1, p. 643).

Those who remained constructed what defenses they could against the fever. These took on strange and varied forms; bonfires,

FIGURE 1-1

Benjamin Rush

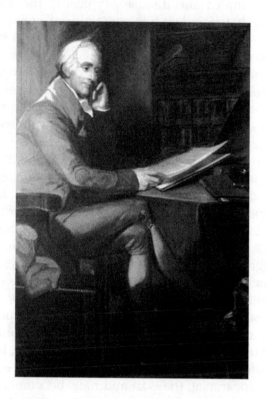

Source: National Library of Medicine.

gunpowder, garlic, tobacco, camphor, vinegar, and antisocial behavior were all a part of the protective arsenal—a most peculiar array by present standards. But 200 years ago, each activity had a rationale.

Outbreaks of yellow fever had been recognized in America since well before the founding of the new republic. The epidemics tended to occur in seaport cities, particularly along the southeast coast. Philadelphia itself had experienced the disease as far back as the time when William Penn first founded the colony. The last major epidemic had been in 1762, and many citizens, including Rush, remembered the devastation it had wrought. From August through December of that year, the death toll mounted daily, reaching as many as 20 each day. Those who had survived that autumn 30 years ago remembered yellow fever well.

It is an unpleasant disease. Typically, the illness begins benignly enough; the patient first complains of a general weariness and weakness—symptoms common to the flu or a host of other unremarkable illnesses. But in a matter of only a few hours this situation can change dramatically. As the disease progresses, there comes a sense of chilliness; a dull pain and giddiness in the head; and an oppressive weight and stricture about the breast, particularly in the region of the heart, as if the space were too narrow for its pulsations. The body temperature rises, there is a pounding headache, and pernicious vomiting ensues. Pains in the muscles of the abdomen and back extend through the arms and legs and cause considerable distress. The skin is flushed, the tongue is dry; the breath becomes foul; the heart races. To this list of symptoms is added almost complete prostration; the body is sapped of strength and incapable of performing many of its normal functions. And so goes the progress of the illness for the first three days.

For some fever sufferers there occurs a temporary respite. The fever falls and symptoms abate. In some instances, recovery follows. For most people with yellow fever, however, things get much worse. Fever and pains return, accompanied by far more alarming symptoms. Vomiting increases, producing ominous, black, "coffee grounds" material. The eyes are bloodshot and the face takes a cadaverous appearance, the skin and nails become a deep yellow color. There is bleeding from the eyes, the nose, the mouth, the bladder. The pulse and blood pressure fall, speech becomes slurred, movements uncoordinated, and the hands tremulous. Red bruises stain the skin. For 20% of victims, death follows, usually about 5 to 8 days after the attack begins. For those who survive, the ordeal typically is concluded in about 2 weeks.

The cause of such a disease and means by which it spread were of great concern, and of considerable controversy. Opinion was strongly divided. Rush led a group that believed that yellow fever had its origins locally, in the decaying organic matter, the filth of the Philadelphia streets. The city's rotting animal carcasses, open sewers, and mounds of festering refuse produced *miasmas*, toxic vapors that poisoned the air. Rush believed that these miasmas combined with predisposing conditions in the body—human failings such as excessive labor or exercise, intemperance, overheating, overcooling, debilitating passions, or violent emotions—to cause disease.

The notion that a disordered atmosphere is responsible for illness is easy to appreciate. The foul smells that accompany decaying animal and vegetable refuse can certainly induce a physical response. Just smelling such decay could make one sick to one's stomach. The coffee that lay rotting on Ball's wharf was a perfect example. As the foul emanations from the dock drifted from the waterfront, in the thick summer heat, the oppressive smell was an obvious sign of an unhealthy atmosphere. Many years of human experience had created linkages between such perturbations in the environment and disease.

As far back as the fifth century B.C., Hippocrates had written of "airs, waters, and places" that predisposed men to disease. "Hot winds cause poor appetite, derangement of the digestive organs, flabby physique; in women they lead to fluxes and barrenness; in children, to asthma, epilepsy, and convulsions; in men, to dysentery, diarrhea, and ague with pleurisy and pneumonia rare. Cold winds make men sinewy, spare and costive; they conduce to pleurisies and acute diseases." Hippocrates goes on to note that cold and frosty waters are responsible for colds and sore throats, while marshy stagnant water is associated with large, stiff spleens and hard, thin, hot stomachs and an illness known as "quartan fever" (3). Indeed, the condition that was associated with the large spleens, recurrent fevers, and the stagnant atmosphere of low-lying swamps became known as "mal-aria"—bad air. There will be more about this topic later.

It also had been long observed that disease occurs more frequently in neighborhoods where filth is rampant and noxious smells abound. Crowded, impoverished, unsanitary neighborhoods of cities are breeding grounds for killers such as typhoid, typhus, and cholera. The creation of causal connections that link the burden of disease to the sensory assaults that are rampant in the stinking slums has obvious appeal. Miasmas make sense as purveyors of disease. Such explanations are a bit too simplistic, as we shall discover later on, but Rush had been convinced. The facts that epidemics such as yellow fever spread so rapidly, often appearing in multiple locations at the same time, argued for an efficient airborne spread. How else could disease appear in households where doors were locked and shutters barred except by unseen evil clouds that seeped in between the cracks?

Opposing Rush's views were *contagionists*, men who were convinced that yellow fever had its origins outside of Philadelphia: The disease was foreign; it had been imported to the city. The source was obvious, they maintained. Since the end of July refugees, fleeing a slave revolt on the island of Santo Domingo in the Caribbean, had been pouring into the city. Ship after ship had spilled its cargo of wretched exiles onto Philadelphia's streets. They were ragged and many were sick. These people had brought the disease with them. The onset of yellow fever in the city coincided exactly with the first influx of refugees. Moreover, it had begun in the precise section of the docks where the immigrants had disembarked. Hadn't some of them been among the first victims identified? These facts were strong evidence as far as contagionists were concerned that the disease was human in its origin and human in its spread. People from outside the city had brought in the plague, and it was being transmitted, not by malevolent vapors, but by contact, from person to person. The view that the disease was imported placed blame for the trouble on outsiders and absolved the city from the burden of responsibility for its own misery.

The theory that one held, whether as miasmatist or contagionist, influenced the approach to stopping the disease. For miasmatists, combating impure air was the essential strategy. For contagionists, it was a matter of minimizing contact between the sick and the well.

Miasmatists, believing the disease was of local origin and born of decay, wanted to clean the city. They argued the necessity of ridding Philadelphia of the refuse and decay that breed foul air. Their strategy was to remove the animal remains, sweep away the heaps of garbage, wash the streets of sewage, and eliminate the putrefying coffee on the docks. They also wanted to purify the tainted atmosphere. That was where the bonfires and the gunpowder came in. Many were convinced that the miasmas could be burned away or that exploding gunpowder had a purifying effect, perhaps by frightening the evil air. It became a battle of pollutants, the familiar smoke driving away the foreign and dangerous miasmas. These approaches had their liabilities, however. The bonfires posed such danger to nearby homes that their risk outweighed putative benefits and prompted the mayor and city council to order that the fires cease. The gunpowder too, was a mixed blessing. Whatever its salutary effects in purifying the atmosphere, they were offset by the unsettling noise of the discharging muskets. The strategy fell from favor.

The less extreme, personal measures Rush had observed in the market makes sense if one believes that disease wafts on the air. The vinegar, the camphor, the garlic, and the cigar smoke all become means to fend off vapors. Each substance produces a friendly, local "atmosphere" to neutralize the larger, malevolent one.

If one believes contagion is the root of the problem, then avoiding contact with the sick is paramount. Several responses are possible. At the personal level, minimizing exposure through personal contacts seems prudent. Thus, the lack of social graces, the absent handshakes, the avoidance of strangers, the empty market all reflect strategies to avoid contact with those who might be harboring disease. Many citizens of Philadelphia, uncertain which camp to join, combined approaches and resorted to any mix of measures they thought might help, including deserting the city altogether. Even Rush himself, though a staunch miasmatist, was taking no chances. He kept his wife and youngest children off in the safer climes of New Jersey, apart from the infected city and its potentially contagious citizens. He advised others to do the same.

For the politicians and government officials, the spreading epidemic presented a special quandary. Should they stay at their posts and do their duty, or flee and live to "fight another day"? The state legislature waffled over what to do. Finally, they conceded that their debates were doing little to combat the spreading fever. On September 5, in response to the governor's admonition that ships were still arriving from the West Indies and importing the contagion, they acted. In rapid succession, they passed a quarantine bill to prevent further importations of disease, granted the governor emergency powers for as long as the epidemic lasted, and adjourned. The quarantine came far too late. By the time the legislature had responded, yellow fever had the city firmly in its grasp. In fact, the only measurable consequences of any regulations restricting passage proved detrimental to Philadelphians. Many who had fled the city to seek refuge in neighboring towns were turned away for fear they were bringing the plague with them, being further induced with tar and feathers.

Rush completed his letter to Julia, cataloging the deaths of neighbors and friends and making the ominous observation that "so universal is the contagion in our city that you meet no one in the street who has not a yellow eye and a dilated pupil" (1, p. 670). Yet, in spite all these travails, he nurtured a surprising sense of hope—even a twinge of exhilaration in the midst of his exhaustion. For, after extreme frustration and failure, after losing more patients than he saved, he had made a discovery—a therapeutic revelation that he believed could save the city.

His earliest approaches to treating yellow fever had been conventional. He had employed mild stimulants: tonics, teas, infusions of bark, as one would do to support a system weakened by fever. He had tried wines and brandies; he attempted to rouse the system by wrapping the body in blankets dipped in warm vinegar. He had buckets of cold water thrown over patients. He had applied ointments and blistering agents to the limbs and neck. Nothing had proved effective. He reckoned that only 3 out of every 13 patients recovered, and those, he thought, might have "recovered much sooner had the cure been trusted to nature" (2, p. 125). Patient after patient, like Mrs. LaMaigre, had turned yellow and died. His despair had deepened.

Then, late one evening at the very end of August, he had "ransacked his library" poring over every book that dealt with yellow fever. Suddenly, he recalled a manuscript that had been given to him by Benjamin Franklin just before the latter's death. And there it was. Right before him, in his own library, lay the answer he had been seeking. The paper, written 50 years earlier by Dr. Mitchell, a physician from Virginia, contained the revelation. Rush had been all wrong in his approach. He had been using stimulants; the barks, the tonics, the wine, assuming the body needed supportive care. In fact, the very opposite was required. Rush had been guilty of assisting nature when he should have been opposing her. He was being meek when boldness was essential. The next morning he began a new approach. For his very first patient he prescribed 10 grains of a chloride of mercury compound called calomel and 15 of a cathartic herb that came from a Mexican tuber known as jalap—three times the normal dose. The patient was then bled. A vein was opened in the left arm and 8 ounces of blood—twice the usual amount—was collected in a pewter bowl. (See Figure 1-2.) Once the calomel and jalap did their work, purging the digestive tract from stem to stern, another bleeding was prescribed. This treatment was followed the next day by more calomel and jalap. Over the ensuing several days there were 5 more bleedings and 5 more purgings. In all, the patient lost 3 pints of blood, the entire contents of his gastrointestinal

FIGURE 1-2

Bloodletting

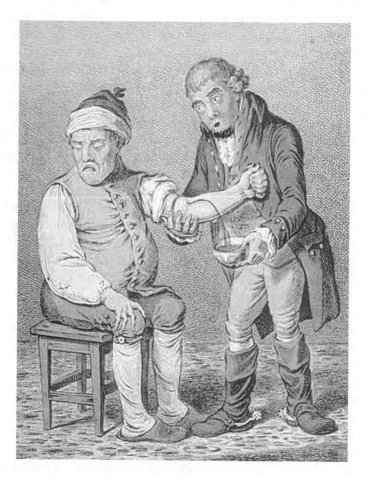

Source: From an etching by Gillray, National Library of Medicine.

tract, and any shreds of dignity. But he survived. Rush was triumphant.

The cure was all so simple, so logical. And Rush had been so slow to see it. Restore balance by depletion, not stimulation; diminish, don't excite; attack the illness, don't mollify nature. It seems a strange approach, but, again, some background is required. Most of us, accustomed to current therapeutics, are oriented to think about specific diseases and specific remedies. Strep throat is a defined illness, caused by the streptococcus germ, that is successfully treated with penicillin. Diabetes, a disease with symptoms caused by high blood sugar due to lack of insulin, can be treated by supplying that missing hormone. High blood pressure and elevated cholesterol, which place individuals at high risk for stroke and heart attack, can be lowered by specific medications. Inflamed appendices cause abdominal pain that is relieved by the surgical removal of the offending tissue. Chest pain resulting from clogged arteries can be alleviated by threading tiny catheters with expandable balloons into the arteries of the heart. And so it goes.

But the concept of specificity was not the rule in Rush's time. It would be another 25 to 30 years before doctors in Paris would begin to carefully examine postmortem specimens and correlate abnormalities in particular organs with patients' clinical complaints. Identification of the tiny germs that would launch the microbiologic revolution lay 90 years in the future. There were some clusters of symptoms and signs that occurred with sufficient consistency that they acquired identity as particular diseases—the characteristic rashes of measles and smallpox, for example, or the painful, swollen joints of gout. However, most illnesses were seen as a problem of a constitution gone astray, the body's usual equilibrium out of balance—too much of one thing or too little of another. And the principle objective of therapeutics was to restore that balance.

Again, one returns to the Greeks who promoted the idea that four bodily fluids or humors are the critical elements of health and disease. These four humors—blood, phlegm, black bile, and yellow bile—enjoy a state of perfect equilibrium in health. When their balance is disrupted, illness ensues. Excesses or deficiencies of the particular humors have predictable consequences. Consider fever, for example. The patient is flushed, the skin is hot and dry, the heart rate rapid. Everything points to an overexcited circulatory system, an excess of blood. Or, consider the congestion that comes with respiratory diseases such as colds and pneumonia. They're caused by too much phlegm. For those afflicted with melancholy or depression, black bile is in clear excess. Each of the humors was associated with one of the four elementary properties of the universe: hot, cold, moist, and dry. And so it fit into a larger pseudoscientific view of the world. Blood was hot and moist; phlegm, cold and moist; black bile, cold and dry; and yellow bile, hot and dry. This conception was consistent with the larger, grander plan. It was a system that had survived hundreds of years.

By the 18th century, however, modifications were being proposed. In Scotland, Rush's mentor, Cullen, was advocating a *solidest* as opposed to *humoral* concept of disease. Cullen theorized that it was the nervous system and its stimulus on muscles of the body that arbitrated health and disease. Illness was not a matter of humoral imbalance but of excessive laxity or tension in the solid tissues. In Cullen's view, fever was caused, not by too much blood, but by an overstimulation of blood vessels, an excitation that caused too much blood to flow and produced the flushing, heat, and accelerated heart rate.

Rush took things a step further. Whereas Cullen decided there were a variety of fevers and, in fact, developed an elaborate system to classify a vast array of illness, Rush was determined to simplify the theory of disease. Rather than embrace his predecessor's dichotomist notions of laxity and tension, of debility and overstimulation, Rush decided that *all* fevers were caused by "morbid excitement" of the blood vessels. In fact, all fevers, he decided, were actually a single entity and were produced by excessive, convulsive spasms of the arteries. Eventually he came upon the notion that not only fevers but all illness could be attributed to abnormal capillary tensions. At one point, he announced to his students that there was really "only one disease in the world."

His unitary theory of disease was defended by clever use of analogies, one scientific and one theological. It makes no more sense, he said, to consider multiple disease mechanisms than to think water, ice, and steam are different elements or that there is more than one God. These were clever arguments. For what learned person could dispute that water, ice, and vapor are all the same compound or suggest that a pantheon existed? When colleagues challenged that several different types of fever were extant in Philadelphia, Rush exploded: "We have but *one*, we cannot have but *one* fever in town.... We might as well talk of two suns or two moons shining upon our globe as of two different kinds of fevers now in our city" (1, p. 683).

The overexcitement and vascular spasms produced not only the flushed, hot skin and rapid pulse of yellow fever but created inner mischief as well. After reading Mitchell's manuscript, Rush decided that the excess stimulation worked adversely on the bowels, creating "obstruction of the liver" and causing internal "putrefaction." Thus the remedies he invoked. To open the obstructed liver and cleanse the gastrointestinal tract, he employed calomel and jalep. Each had a direct, toxic effect on the intestinal tract and caused a violent evacuation of the bowels. Often, not content that the visible signs of purging were sufficient, Rush insisted that the calomel be given until patients displayed excess salivation—a sign of mercury poisoning. Bloodletting was likewise consistent with his theories of disease. Reducing the volume of circulating blood was a direct attack upon the heightened vascular tension. It dampened the overstimulated system. Multiple bouts of bleeding were required, until all evidence of excessive excitement was quelled. Often, this meant repeating the procedure to the point where the patient was quite weak and debilitated. All necessary, Rush claimed, if a cure was to be effected.

Rush believed his "heroic" approach was capable of producing miracles. "Never before did I experience such sublime joy as I now felt in contemplating the success of my remedies," he crowed. "It repaid me for all the toils and studies of my life. The conquest of this formidable disease was not the effect of accident, nor of the application of a single remedy; but it was the triumph of a principle of medicine" (2, p. 131). The greatest miracle was that any patients survived his ministrations. His convictions brooked little tolerance for the ignorance displayed by colleagues who were not advocates of his approach. "My labors in combating the disease have been great.... They were successful in 99 cases out of 100," he boasted with numerical authority, " but my principal exertions have been created by the pride, ignorance, and prejudices of my medical brethren. From the dull Dr. Kuhn down to the volatile Dr. B. Duffield ..., they have all combined to oppose, to depreciate, and even to slander the new remedies" (1, p. 681).

But as forcefully as Rush argued his ideas of the origins and spread of yellow fever and as vigorously as he promoted and defended his therapies, one crucial element was missing. Nothing was ever tested. Rush never challenged his theories with experiment. To be certain, he did make note of his successes. But though he wrote extensively and recorded many of his thoughts in diaries, letters, newspapers, and books, he never systematically documented his case records so others could reliably learn from his experience. He relied entirely on anecdotes, and those were carefully selected to support his new-found cure. Each patient who survived was a testament to the new remedy. Those who died were dismissed as seeking aid too late in the course of their illness for the cure to take effect. There were no records of the details of timing, dose, and outcome. Rush's claim that 99 of 100 treatments had succeeded had no data to support it.

Rush was not alone in this documentation. Few physicians practicing at the end of the 18th century considered collecting information on the experiences of their patients as a means to test the efficacy of their therapeutics. Medical practice was driven entirely by theory, and the thought that experiment should inform and even modify practice was unthinkable. Educated physicians wrote and debated endlessly their theories of cause and therapy. But the idea that such theories could be tested, as Joseph Priestley had done when he discovered oxygen, or Franklin had when he lofted his kite toward the heavens, was not considered. In fact, those who relied on experience and experimented with therapeutics without a clear basis in theory were dismissed as quacks or "empirics." The science of medicine lagged woefully behind the physical sciences as the century drew to a close.

It was no small irony, that, though Rush failed to provide numeric evidence of the benefits of his therapy, numbers were marshaled against him. A major detractor and vocal enemy, William Cobbett, examined the yellow fever mortality lists to discredit Rush and his "heroic" therapeutics.

Cobbett was a disaffected Englishman who immigrated to America in 1792 to escape the tyranny and corruption he saw pervading his homeland. Cobbett settled in Philadelphia, where he set up a bookselling, publishing, and print shop on Second Street, across from Christ Church. (See Figure 1-3.) But his love affair with America and her new democracy was short-lived. He rapidly grew disenchanted with the New World, finding that dream and reality were far apart. Where he had hoped to find "a land of liberty, virtue, and simplicity," he, instead, experienced "exactly the contrary of what I expected…. The land is bad, rocky…. The seasons are detestable…; The people, worthy of the country—(a) cheating, sly, roguish gang" (4, p. 10). Cobbett had already established himself as an acerbic critic and pamphleteer in England, and barbs against those things that displeased him in America soon showered from

FIGURE 1-3

Philadelphia in the 1790s. Second Street Looking North from Market Street towards Christ Church. Cobbett's Publishing and Printing Shop was Across from the Church

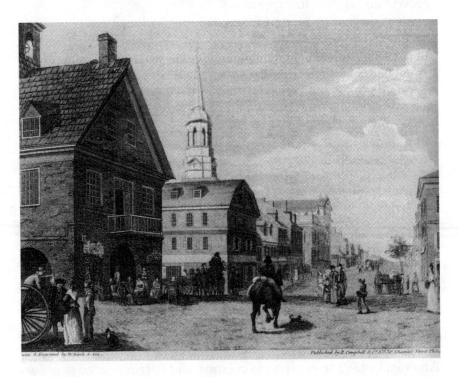

Source: From an engraving by Birch, Library of Congress.

his pen. He adopted the appropriately prickly nom-de-plume of Peter Porcupine and published much of his invective in a pamphlet he called *Porcupine's Gazette*.

Benjamin Rush was high on the list of things that displeased Cobbett, and the critic pilloried the doctor in series of pamphlets called *The Rush-Light*. "The loathsome subject now before me, is not taken up by choice but from a sense of duty" (4, p. 228). Of particular annoyance were Rush's drastic therapeutics and the arrogance Rush displayed in promoting them. Peter Porcupine was not the only one to criticize Rush for the excessive bleeding and purging techniques. But he was the most outspoken. Ultimately, Peter Porcupine's quills were his undoing. Rush sued him for liable. After a trial in which the selection of the judge and jury tipped the scales of justice heavily in favor of Rush, Cobbett was assessed the ruinous fine of $5000. Further embittered and now destitute, he fled back to England.

Cobbett's numerical counter to Rush's claim that bleeding and purging saved lives was based on the daily counts of yellow fever deaths. Cobbett observed that Rush had begun promoting his therapeutic approach on September 12, when the death rate stood at 33 per day. He reasoned that, if the Rush approach were beneficial, there should be a leveling and then decline in deaths over subsequent weeks. This, he demonstrates, was not the case, as Figure 1-4 shows. The daily toll rises steadily from early September to the middle of October, peaking at over 100 deaths each day. "Thus you see," sneered Cobbett, "that though the fever was on the 12th of September reduced to a level with a common cold [Rush's boast]; though the lancet was continually unsheathed; though Rush and his subalterns were ready at every call, the deaths did actually increase." The sarcasm continued: "Astonishing obstinacy! Perverse Philadelphians! Not withstanding there was a man in your city who could have healed you with a touch you continued to die! Not withstanding that precious purges were advertised at every corner, and were brought even to your doors and bedsides …, still you persisted in dying" (5). It was an argument of some persuasion. And Rush offered no numbers to counter the attack.

The closest Rush came to employing data to support his claims was when he predicted the end of the epidemic on the basis of a change in the weather. Like others of his time, he was fascinated with the relationship between weather and disease. With his staunch

FIGURE 1-4

Deaths from Yellow Fever in Philadelphia, September 10 to November. 9, 1793.

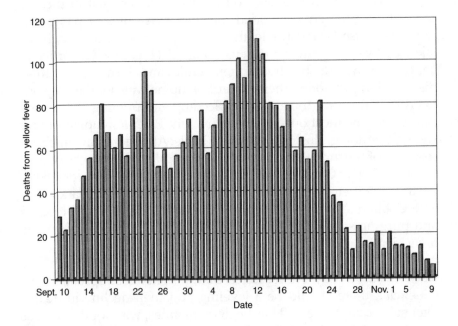

Source: Based on Rush, *Medical Inquiries and Observations* (2).

belief in miasmas, it is not surprising that he was convinced that tracking weather and atmospheric patterns would help explain the waxing and waning of illness. On the chilly evening of September 18, when he had written his wife of his illness, Rush had hoped that the sudden influx of cool weather might diminish the progress of the outbreak. In previous epidemics new cases had dropped dramatically soon after the season turned cold and the autumn frosts cleared the pestilent air. It was not to be. The warm, dry weather had returned and persisted through late September and into October. The disease had gone on unabated, tallying a death toll of as many as 100 Philadelphians a day.

Then, in mid-October, a cold front from the north brought in rain and a sudden drop of temperature into the low 30s. "On the fifteenth of October, it pleased God to alter the state of the air," Rush wrote.

"The clouds at last dropped health in showers of rain, which continued during the whole day, and which were succeeded for several nights by cold and frost. The effects of this change in the weather appeared first in the sudden diminution of the sick, for the deaths continued for a week afterward to be numerous, but they were persons who had been confined before, or on the day in which the change had taken place in the weather" (2, p. 98).

The right-hand side of Figure 1-4 supports his observation. A sharp decline in deaths begins about 1 week after the change in weather. But how certain can we be that it is the "showers of rain" that are responsible for the therapeutic effect? Could there be other factors that accompany the cool weather that are more directly related to the drop in deaths? We will take up these questions later.

Use of *statistics*, of the assembled enumeration of health events, was in its nascence in the 18th century. Efforts to collect *mortality* figures to learn something of the health of populations can be traced to the 1660s, when an Englishman named John Graunt published *Bills of Mortality*, which catalogued the deaths for London. But sustained efforts to gather such data had yet to take hold. In the new republic, some mortality data were to be had, but they were sparse and of modest reliability, at best. Most were gathered by church sextons as reports of burials. These collections were highly variable in consistency and quality, and they were far from universally available. The causes of death recorded followed no standard classification schemes.

This lack of interest in data was consistent with the philosophy of *rationalism* that dominated medical thought at the time. Practice was driven by theory rather than by experience. Physicians were far more influenced by opinion, ideology, and prejudice than by facts, collected or otherwise. So practices we consider as standard today, such as trials that compare treatments head to head among groups of human subjects to see which works best, were not considered. Instead, each physician proceeded independently, selecting therapies based on polemics rather than on scientific principles—not a situation that best served the public's health.

We have come far since then. Medicine and public health have become disciplines with scientific cores. We have gained much sophistication in collecting, counting, and assembling health data. Research methods have been developed that provide a basis for

making decisions about which medical treatments are truly beneficial to patients and which preventive approaches will actually
ward off disease.

The journey to where we are today, with our remarkable
understanding of the causes of disease and impressive array of
therapeutic successes, is the substance of the succeeding chapters.
That endeavor has not been easy. The study of humans is difficult.
It makes working with chemicals or electricity or white mice seem
simple. There is variability, uncertainty, and inconsistency at every
turn. People are living, moving targets—changing locations, habits,
opinions, activities, diets, and feelings. Information they give you
at one time may change at the next. What works for some people,
doesn't help others. The path has not been direct. Progress has been
halting, and large temporal gaps are evident. Experiences of the
past don't always appear to influence those working in the present.
But the stories that make up the journey are intriguing and informative. They are rich in their human dimension as well as instructive for the scientific issues they raise.

The epidemic of yellow fever in Philadelphia was over by
mid-November of 1793. The final tally of lives reached over 4000,
about 10% of Philadelphia's population. It was, however, not the
last the city was to see of the disease. Yellow fever revisited the following summer and almost every year until 1805. Through these
repeated invasions, Rush held fervently to his beliefs about transmission and treatment, contributing more to controversy than to
clarity. He went on to be remembered as one of America's most
influential physicians. In fairness, his legacy is based more on his
early work in mental health than on his bleeding of yellow fever
victims. Yet, Rush came tantalizingly close to being a hero rather
than a goat in the yellow fever saga. He missed by a hairsbreadth
a stunning contribution to the understanding of the disease. His
observation that the yellow fever abated soon after the autumn
frost was quite correct. Within it lay a critical clue to solving the
mystery of the illness. But Rush thought the cold weather simply
cleansed the air of miasmas. He failed to consider other changes
that accompany frost as well; the role, for example, in the life cycle
of a common insect pest. That, it turned out, was a discovery that
would have to wait for another 100 years.

REFERENCES

1. Butterfield LH, ed. *Letters of Benjamin Rush*. Princeton: Princeton University Press; 1951.
2. Rush B. *Medical Inquiries and Observations*. Vol. 3, 4th ed. Philadelphia: Griggs & Dickinsons; 1815.
3. Chadwick J, Mann WN. *The Medical Work of Hippocrates*. Oxford: Blackwell Scientific; 1950.
4. Cobbett W, Wilson DA. *Peter Porcupine in America: Pamphlets on Republicanism and Revolution*. Ithaca: Cornell University Press; 1994.
5. Peter Porcupine. *The Rush-Light*. New York: William Cobbett; 1800.

Doctors and Ministers: Smallpox in Boston, 1721

It was a disordered time. Smallpox was raging in the colonial town of Boston. The outbreak had begun in the spring. At first there were only a few cases, but over the summer the outbreak grew so that by the autumn of 1721 more than 100 deaths were being tallied every week—in a town of only 10,000 people. Commerce was in disarray. The flow of essential goods into the town had been drastically curtailed. Fearing for their lives, tradesmen had stopped delivering butter, grain, and firewood to the contaminated community. Families with the means were abandoning the town, retreating to the relative safety of the countryside. It was a struggle for survival and a time for Boston's leaders to rally the citizenry, to hold the town together.

Instead, a second struggle was taking place. A war of words and wills was being contested between the town's clergymen and its doctors. It was a vitriolic debate that centered on a controversial new medical technique that was intended to protect the public against the ravages of smallpox. The procedure was called inoculation. It involved the direct transfer of infectious matter from a pustule on a patient in the active throes of smallpox to a healthy individual. This inoculation, it was believed, would create a mild form of the disease in the recipient, illness that had little chance of causing death. The benefit of brief indisposition would be lifelong resistance to smallpox thereafter. It was an extraordinary idea, a true medical breakthrough. But the approach was not universally embraced. It had created vocal camps of supporters and detractors. The lines were not drawn as one would have anticipated, however. The roles of the antagonists were strangely reversed. In support of inoculation were the town's clergy—in strong opposition, its doctors.

The medical men, the men of science, opposed inoculation on religious principle. They were appalled at the idea of purposely infecting healthy individuals with a devastating disease like small-pox. It was, they contended, a potent affront to God. Firm adherents to Puritan notions of the direct relationship between human sin and divine punishment, they believed the disease was righteous retribution for human failings. Mankind deserved the punishment and the only proper response was fasting and repentance—seeking God's forgiveness. Any human activity that interfered with the divine order of things represented sacrilege. They decried the practice of, "trusting more the extra groundless machinations of men than to our Preserver" (1, p. 57).

Surprisingly, the ministers advocated for inoculation. Though equally committed to obedience to divine design, they were convinced that true virtue lay in preventing the grave human suffering created by smallpox. They argued that inoculation *was* part of God's plan. The procedure was given to man by God just as were other medical treatments. They wrote that the procedure should be accepted "with all the thankfulness and joy as the gracious discovery of a kind providence to mankind for that end," and added, "do we not in the use of all means depend on God's blessing?...What hand or art of man is there in this operation more than in bleeding, blistering and a score more things in medical use?" (1, p. 57). A strange situation indeed, physicians opposing a medical procedure on religious grounds; the ministers answering with a medical argument.

The chief proponent of the new procedure was the Reverend Cotton Mather, a prominent Puritan minister. Mather was 58 years old when the inoculation debate began. Widely considered to be one of the colony's most intelligent men, he was also known to be opinionated, arrogant, and quarrelsome. The precocious son of another eminent man of the cloth, he was capable of translating English sermons into Latin at the age of 11 and had completed Harvard by the age of 15. He was ordained in his father's church when he was 23 (see Figure 2-1).

FIGURE 2-1

Cotton Mather

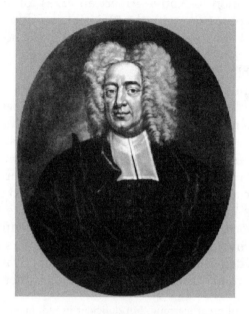

Source: From a painting by Pelham, National Library of Medicine.

Mather was not a stranger to controversy. He had been at the center of squabbles over church doctrine and was identified as a ringleader in a political rebellion against England's appointed colonial governor.

His chief notoriety, however, had come from his association with the Massachusetts witch trials. Though not an active participant in the proceedings, his writings on the "Wonders of the Invisible World," in which he supported the trials and proclaimed that the devil was playing havoc in New England, were published at a moment when the prosecutions were becoming highly unpopular. His reputation was greatly damaged.

Mather's conviction that supernatural forces were at work in New England and his insistence that the world of demons was real appear in surprising contrast to his otherwise analytic mind. He was one of the country's first scientists, elected to fellowship in England's academic Royal Society for his scientific observations on a variety of the New World's natural phenomena. His reports ranged from descriptions of rattlesnakes and hummingbirds to plant hybridization to Native American cures for syphilis. At the same time his obsession with the "invisible world" prompted him to keep several "possessed" young women in his home to observe firsthand the manifestations of their torment: the fits of choking, the spells of blindness, the screaming discourses with "the dark one." The culmination of all this came with a personal visitation from a benevolent angel bedecked in a shining white robe, and magnificent tiara, with wings sprouting from the shoulders.

Opposing Mather and other influential Boston clergymen who shared his support of inoculation were all but one of the town's 10 doctors. They were led by a vigorous and vituperative young Scottish physician who had only recently immigrated to the colonies. His name was William Douglass. Douglass was the best educated of Boston's doctors and the town's most self-confident. He had studied medicine in the important European centers of Edinburgh, Paris, and Leyden. But the quality of his training was not sufficient to endear him to his fellow citizens. One biographer noted:

> He was a man of great learning, but deficient in judgment, prudence and correct taste; yet he assumed the task of animadverting upon the actions and characteristics of others, filling the newspapers with political essays fraught with sarcastic remarks upon the magistrates, the clergy, and physicians, and the people of New England. (2, pp. 255–325)

Opinions were strong, and the debate, contentious. There was one point, however on which everyone agreed. Smallpox was a disease to avoid. It is an ordeal that begins, like many illnesses, with a fever and a general sense of malaise. Accompanying the fever is a splitting headache and, often, severe pains in the back. At this juncture, there is nothing to distinguish the disease from many of its contagious counterparts. Typically, after two or three days, the fever falls to normal, hinting at recovery. But the respite is a cruel hoax, for at this juncture the illness begins in earnest. A rash begins— initially as small red spots on the forearms and face. More troubling lesions erupt in the mouth and throat, making swallowing painful. The small red spots soon grow to small, tense vesicles, or blebs. At first, these blebs contain clear fluid, but then they become cloudy and pustular. The rash becomes aggressive and within a day or two overspreads most of the body's surface, including palms of the hands and soles of the feet. The fever also returns. The second week of illness is worse. Patients suffer greatly. A contemporary of Mather describes this stage quite graphically:

> Purple Spots, the bloody and parchment Pox, Hemorahages of Blood at the Mouth, Nose, Fundament, and Privities; Ravings and Deliriums; Convulsions, and other Fits; violent inflammations and Swellings in the Eyes and Throat; so that they cannot see, or scarcely breathe, or swallow any thing, to keep them from starving. Some looking as black as the Stock, others as white as a Sheet; in some, the Pock runs into Blisters, and the Skin stripping off, leaves the Flesh raw.... Some have been fill'd with loathsome Ulcers; others have had deep, and fistulous Ulcers in their Bodies, or in their Limbs or Joints, with Rottenness of the Ligaments and Bones: Some who live are Cripples, others Idiots, and many blind all their Days. (3, pp. 337–338)

Most who succumb die during this interval. For the more fortunate, healing begins after about 2 weeks of torture. The skin lesions form crusts, then scabs, which eventually separate to reveal regenerating skin. For unfortunate patients there are residual scars. The single benefit to the ordeal is that once endured, the illness never returns. Survivors are immune for the remainder of their lives.

Smallpox has a long history of tormenting humans. Our earliest evidence of the disease comes from the Middle East; Egyptian mummies dating from 1500 to 1000 B.C. have visible signs of what appear to be pox marks. The well-preserved remains of Ramses V, who died in 1157 B.C., display an array of marks that have a characteristic distribution over the face and arms. Microscopic examinations of skin samples support the diagnosis. Written documents from India, China, and Greece suggest the disease was known before the time of Christ in these regions as well.

During the 3 millennia between Ramses V and Cotton Mather, smallpox compiled a legacy of misery and death. It killed kings, brought armies to submission, decimated native populations, and humbled empires. Regal victims included Queen Mary II of Scotland, Joseph I of Austria, Louis I of Spain, Peter II of Russia, and Louis XV of France. Queen Elizabeth I of England was among its most famous survivors, but one who carried the scars left by the disease with her for a lifetime. Smallpox was a far more decisive force in the Spanish conquest of Mexico than all the military prowess of the conquistadors. By some estimates one-half of the native population of Mexico had perished within the year after Spanish ships brought smallpox to Vera Cruz in 1520 A.D. (4, 206–207) (see Figure 2-2).

With this history of suffering, it should be no surprise that any measure that promised relief from smallpox would be a thrilling prospect. Such was Cotton Mather's view. His introduction to the procedure, known as implantation, or inoculation, came from an unexpected source. A grateful congregation had presented their minister with a black servant named Onesimus, a man who had been brought from the northwestern corner of Africa in 1706. In questioning the man about his previous health, Mather asked Onesimus if he had ever experienced the smallpox. The answer provided was a paradoxical "yes and no." When Mather probed, he found that the servant had undergone a rite in his native country in which he had been intentionally injected with pus from a smallpox victim. The idea was to avoid contracting more serious disease naturally. Mather, who relished and collected unusual scientific anecdotes, packed the story away in his store of medical curiosities.

Then, in 1716, a physician, who had recently arrived in the colonies from Scotland, and carried letters of introduction to the

FIGURE 2-2

Aztec Smallpox Victim

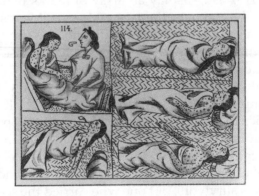

Source: Codice Florentino.

influential minister, lent Mather several volumes of the *Philosophical Transactions of the Royal Society of London*. There, to the Reverend's fascination, was a report from Turkey, of the very protective procedure Onesimus had described years earlier. Mather was exhilarated. He wrote to John Woodward of the Royal Society to detail his servant's story and vowed that when next smallpox struck the colonies, he would persuade Boston's doctors to take up the practice, "If I should live to see the smallpox again enter our city, I would immediately procure a consult of our physicians, to introduce (the) practice" (1, p. 54). The doctor, who loaned the *Transactions* to Mather, was William Douglass.

Five more years passed. Then, in mid-April, several ships from the West Indies sailed into Boston Harbor, past the quarantine station to dock at Long Wharf. One of the ships, HMS *Seahorse*, carried several aboard who were incubating smallpox. It was May 8 when the first case broke out in town. Soon a second was discovered. The town selectman ordered guards be placed to prevent transmission from the infected houses. They ordered the *Seahorse* into quarantine at Bird Island, but it was too late. Pandora's Box was open.

By the end of May the disease had spread. Eight cases had been identified. The quarantine had failed. Mather acted on his promise. On June 6 he wrote to the physicians of Boston, sending them abstracts of accounts of inoculation from the Royal Society. He urged the doctors to read the reports and take up the practice. There was no response. Not a single doctor came forward to challenge smallpox with the exciting new method. Mather despaired. He worried for his flock and for his town. A devoted father, he also worried for his family. He noted in his diary, "I have two children who are liable to the distemper; and I am at a loss about their flying and keeping out of the town." As the smallpox cases grew in number and no advocates for inoculation came forward, he fretted to the diary: "What shall I do? What shall I do with regard onto Sammy [his son]? He comes home when the smallpox begins to spread in the neighborhood; and he is loathe to return unto Cambridge, I must earnestly look up to Heaven for direction" (5, pp. 621–626).

Mather tried again. This time he wrote specifically to Dr. Zabdiel Boylston, pleading with him to take responsibility for the town's deliverance. Boylston, the son of a Boston doctor, had been trained by his father in the apprentice tradition. He was one of 10 doctors in the town and a man of multiple parts. Boylston mingled talents as apothecary, physician, surgeon, tradesman, and naturalist. His small pharmacy sold not only medicinals and surgical implements but also painter's colors and nostrums for growing hair. His surgical achievements included removal of kidney stones and, quite remarkably, a successful mastectomy. He had also achieved some standing as a naturalist, transmitting unusual specimens of American plants, animals, and insects to edify the Royal Society in England.

Boylston rose to Mather's challenge. On June 26, he made two short, parallel incisions on the arm of his own 6-year-old son, Thomas. After wiping away the two thin lines of blood, he placed a small tuft of lint that he had dipped in a vial containing pus from the lesion of a smallpox patient on to the wound. He then covered it with a nutshell so that the inoculum would not be rubbed off by the boy's clothing. Several days passed. Then, 7 days after the procedure had been performed, Thomas began to run a fever. The site on his arm turned red and angry. Pustules developed in a circle around the spot then spread in small numbers over his arm and chest. The fever lasted for 3 days. One week after their first appearance, the pustules began to scab and heal and, by three weeks after the inoculation, the boy was well.

It was a brief, undramatic event. But it did not pass unnoticed. Within a few days after Boylston performed his experiment "an horrid clamor" began (5, p. 628). Not only were Boylston's colleagues alarmed, but Boston's citizenry was aroused in opposition. Mather regarded the uproar as clear evidence of the devil at work. He noted in his diary: "The Destroyer, being enraged at the proposal of anything that may rescue the lives of our poor people from him, has taken a strange possession of the people on this occasion. They rave, they rail, they blaspheme; they talk not only like idiots but also like frantics, and not only the physician who began the experiment, but I also am an object of their fury" (5, p. 632). As the controversy grew over ensuing days, Mather lamented, "the cursed clamor of a people strangely and fiercely possessed of the devil, will probably prevent my saving the lives of my 2 children from the smallpox in the way of transplantation [inoculation]" (5, p. 632).

On July 24 the town selectmen called a meeting. They ignored Boylston's offer to demonstrate the success of his procedure. Instead, they accepted the testimony of a French physician named Dalhonde, who stated, on the basis of his experience in Europe, that inoculation "has proved the death of many persons" and "tends to spread and continue the infection." He also claimed that the procedure was often ineffectual (2, p. 42). The selectmen were persuaded by his testimony. They admonished Boylston and demanded he desist from practicing the procedure further.

Douglass attacked Boylston in the *Boston News-Letter*, characterizing the latter as illiterate and ignorant and blaming him for "mischievous propagating (of) the infection in the most publick [sic] trading place of the Town" (1, p. 57). The ministers leaped to Boylston's defense:

> It was a grief to us the subscribers, among others of your friends in the town, to see Dr. *Boylston* treated so unhandsomely in the letter directed to you last week, and published in your paper. He is a son of the town whom heaven (we all know) has adorn'd with some very peculiar gifts for the service of his country.(6, p. 319)

Boylston persisted. He continued inoculating patients and stirring the coals of controversy. In August, he implanted smallpox on 17 patients including, finally, Sammy, the son of the anxious Mather. There were 31 more innoculees in September, 18 in October. By November, he was up to 104. All this while the epidemic raged. In October, the outbreak peaked, with over 400 deaths recorded. In November mortality was down to 249 and, as winter settled in, the contagion quietly disappeared from Boston. By the time it was over, about half the population had been afflicted; 1 in 7 of those had succumbed to the infection. There had been 842 deaths from smallpox among the 5700 who had acquired the disease.

Though the immediate danger of smallpox had abated, Boylston continued inoculating, albeit at a reduced pace. When, in May, he performed the procedure on Samuel Sewall, his wife, and four others, the town had had enough. The selectmen met and immediately ordered the inoculees into quarantine on Spectacle Island. They again admonished Boylston and extracted his solemn promise to "inoculate no more without the knowledge and approbation of the authority of the town." Legislation was also proposed to regulate inoculation, prohibiting it from any town without the expressed consent of the selectman. Douglass was triumphant:

> Last January Inoculation made a Sort of Exit, like the Infatuation thirty years ago, after several had fallen victims to the mistaken notions of Dr. M–r and other learned clerks concerning Witchcraft. But finding Inoculation in this town, like the Serpents in the Summer, beginning to crawl abroad again the last Week, it was in time, and effectually crushed in the Bud, by Justices, Select-Men, and the unanimous Vote of a general Town-Meeting. (1, p. 62)

But where does the truth lie in all the charges and counter-charges? Was inoculation an evil or a benefit? The continuing quarrel contained several arguments. The first, that has been previously mentioned, was religious. Did man have the right to intervene in the divine order of things? Both sides of the inoculation question could be easily defended, depending on how broadly one considered the divine plan to be. Was punishing human transgression by inflicting smallpox on sinners the extent of divine intent, or did God's plan include, as the ministers claimed, the remedy as well? The dispute is difficult to resolve.

The second issue was a medical one: contagion. Could the practice of inoculation actually contribute to spread of disease and propagation of the epidemic? Opponents claimed this was an obvious risk and that the liabilities of propagating outbreaks of smallpox greatly outweighed any benefits of the procedure. But evidence (either for or against) was difficult to obtain. With naturally occurring smallpox rampant in the town, how could one pinpoint just where or from whom any victim had acquired infection? The apparent consensus that the disease was, in fact, passed from person to person comes as something of a surprise. The disagreements over the cause and spread of illness that existed during Benjamin Rush's time were no less prevalent 70 years earlier. But smallpox was one of the few diseases that almost everyone agreed was spread from person to person. The presentation was so consistent, the rash so characteristic, and the trail of contacts so easy to trace.

Current knowledge confirms these observations. Smallpox is a viral disease. It is caused by a submicroscopic particle of genetic

material encased in a protein and sugar capsule known scientifi-
cally as *Variola major*. A virus by itself is not a living organism. It
survives and replicates only through its parasitic relationship with
living cells. The virus particle attaches to a cell, typically of the respiratory or gastrointestinal tract, and inserts its genetic core into
the interior of its host. There, the strands of genetic material
(known as *nucleic acids*) subvert the cell's information processing
system to their own purposes. The viral genetic material (the
genome) directs the cell to make new viruses. The unwary cell
responds and manufactures new particles that, with ultimate
ingratitude, break from their host and destroy it.

That smallpox is contagious is now well established. The
virus invades its host by way of the respiratory tract. Viral particles made airborne by a cough or a sneeze are briefly suspended
in the air. These are inhaled by people in proximity to those with
illness and lodge on membranes in the nose and throat. The particles penetrate the tissues, then migrate to lymph nodes, where
they multiply. Released from the lymph nodes into the blood, they
are transported to the skin and back to the cells of the mouth and
throat. Once lodged in these locations, they initiate the spots, pustules, and the sores within the mouth. These lesions contain the
viral particles, and they become the source of continuing transmission. A cough or sneeze from the newly infected nose or throat
creates a new cloud of virus droplets ready to be inhaled by a fresh
victim.

In theory, the inoculated virus could be spread and could create epidemics where there were none before. In fact, this did not
occur. For reasons still not certain, the virus acquired by implantation was less harmful than when acquired by the usual respiratory
route. Introduction through the skin dampened its destructive
powers. Most illness that resulted was limited to pustules around
the inoculation site. Signs of serious systemic spread were infrequent, and the quantity of virus present in the respiratory tract
available to be dispersed by cough or sneeze was low. The fear that
inoculation could propagate or create new epidemics was over-
drawn. But neither Boylston nor Douglass knew this.

The rancor that continued more than a year did little to alter
opposing opinions or enlighten a fearful public. Invective held
dominion over science. Almost no attention was paid to the most

fundamental questions, "Did inoculation actually work? Did it protect against death from smallpox?" It was not until some months
after the heat had subsided that the issue was examined. Boylston
had inoculated a total of 247 people. But not all of his experiments
had met with success. Six of his patients died. The deaths, of
course, provided fodder for critics. Boylston had deliberately
infected people in the expectation they would be spared the serious
consequences of smallpox and, instead, he had precipitated their
deaths. These were not outcomes to appease adversaries, and they
were seized upon to discredit the procedure. Yet both Mather and
Boylston were savvy enough to understand that 6 inoculation
deaths did not mean failure.

The question was not whether inoculation was completely
safe, whether deaths could be avoided altogether, but whether outcomes were better after inoculation than when disease was
acquired naturally. This could be answered by a straightforward
statistical comparison. With 842 deaths among the 5700 victims of
"natural smallpox," a simple proportion indicates that 14.6, or
almost 15% of cases, died (see Table 2-1). This ratio, the number of
deaths to number of cases, is known as a *case fatality rate*. The same
calculation for inoculated cases yields a case fatality rate of only
2.1%. The rate of death for those contracting natural smallpox
was 7 times greater than for those who received it by inoculation.
It's a compelling bit of arithmetic. It represents the first example

TABLE 2-1

Inoculation Statistics for Boston, 1721

Population	10,700		
Natural Smallpox		*Inoculated Smallpox*	
Cases	5,759	Cases	287
Deaths	842	Deaths	6
Deaths per 100 cases	14.6	Deaths per 100 cases	2.1

*Boylston was responsible for 247 inoculations. Several other physicians contributed the remainder of the cases.
Source: Based on Blake (1), p. 244.

of a scientific, statistical approach to evaluating a public health intervention in North America.

The experiment was to be repeated over the next 45 years, as epidemics of smallpox revisited Boston. Table 2-2 shows data for death rates from naturally acquired and inoculation induced small-pox during subsequent epidemics.

Several points are worth noting. First, the death rates for natu-rally occurring smallpox are remarkably consistent. The case fatality rate ranges between about 10% in 1752 and 18% in the 1764 epi-demic. Case fatality rates for inoculated cases are also similar for the four epidemics, ranging from about 1% to 3%. From the scien-tific point of view, such repetition is encouraging. The *consistency* of results strengthens the evidence that the procedure is beneficial. The advantage for inoculation is seen in four different epidemics occurring at different times and affecting different generations of subjects. The experience of Boylston and Mather does not appear to be a "one time fluke."

It is also of note that the practice of inoculation grew even though resistance continued over the 40-year interval. In the epidemic of 1730 only 400 subjects received smallpox through inoculation against a

TABLE 2-2

Inoculation Statistics for Boston, 1721–1764

	1721	1730	1752	1764
Population	10,700	13,500	15,684	15,500
Natural Smallpox				
Cases	5,759	3,600	5,545	699
Deaths	842	500	539	124
Deaths per 100 cases	14.6	13.9	9.9	17.7
Inoculated Smallpox				
Cases	287	400	2,124	4,977
Deaths	6	12	30	46
Deaths per 100 cases	2.1	3.0	1.4	0.9

Source: Based on Blake (1), p. 244.

background of 3600 naturally occurring cases. Twenty-two years later, in 1752, there were over 2000 inoculations and 5500 natural cases. By 1764 almost 5000 inoculations took place and far exceeded naturally occurring smallpox cases.

Over time the procedure spread to other colonies. In Philadelphia it gained the endorsement of an ex-Bostonian who had been in the thick of the initial controversy. Benjamin Franklin was just a teenage apprentice in his brother's Boston printing shop in 1721. The brother, James, had been an outspoken critic of inoculation. His paper, the *New England Courant*, served as the repository for anti-inoculation invective. But as he matured, Benjamin went over to the other side. By 1736 Franklin had moved to Philadelphia, married, and had a son. The boy contracted smallpox and died. Concerned at rumors that Frankie had died after being inoculated, Franklin wrote to the *Pennsylvania Gazette* to set the record straight:

> Understanding 'tis a current report that my son Francis, who died lately of the smallpox, had it by inoculation; and being desired to satisfy the public in that particular; in as much as some people are, by that report...deterred from having that operation preformed on their children, I do hereby sincerely declare, that he was not inoculated, but received the distemper in the common way of infection. (7, p. 190)

Grief over the fact his son's death might have been avoided had the boy been inoculated turned Franklin to an advocate. Some years later, while in England in 1759, he enlisted the aid of a respected English physician, William Heberden, to collaborate on a pamphlet that would provide basic instructions for the public on performing the procedure. The goal was to make protection from smallpox widely available in "places where it is not easy to procure the assistance of physicians and surgeons" (7, p. 192). Franklin also noted that "the expense of having the operation performed by a surgeon...has been pretty high in some parts of America; and where a common tradesman or artificer has a number in his family to have the distemper, it amounts to more money that he can well spare" (7, p. 196).

Franklin contributed to the data that supported inoculation. Inquiries made of doctors in Philadelphia who practiced the procedure indicated there had been only 4 fatalities among about

800 inoculees. Franklin even gathered similar figures from England, from Dr. Archer, who was the physician to a special smallpox hospital there. His findings are shown in Table 2-3. The case fatality rates for those who were inoculated are less than 1% ($6/1601 = 0.4\%$), far lower than when the disease was "had in the common way" ($1002/3856 = 26\%$) (7, pp. 197–198).

Boylston and Mather and Franklin make a major contribution to the process of determining the efficacy of an intervention. They use the strategy of *comparisons*. They demonstrate that inoculation is successful, by the use of data rather than through the force of philosophy—empiricism rather than rationalism. Their comparison of the case fatality rates is strong evidence. It is a straightforward, powerful argument. Usually 1 in every 7 cases of smallpox ends fatally. But, among those who are inoculated only 2% die from the disease. Simple but elegant. The use of a comparison acknowledges that there is a natural course of a disease in a human population and that a successful intervention must improve upon the usual outcomes. This concept feels quite familiar to us today, but it was not in evidence in the medical thought of colonial times.

The strategy of comparing outcomes of those given interventions to prevent disease with those who acquired disease naturally has become a basic tool for public health and medical research. The technique makes use of what we would call a *natural experiment*. It is an approach that has been a long time in developing, but is still being used to answer questions similar to those posed by the problem

TABLE 2-3

Inoculation Statistics for London Smallpox Hospital, 1758

	Persons
There have been inoculated in this Hospital since its first institution to this day, Dec. 31, 1758	1601
Of which number died	6
Patients who had the smallpox in the common way in this hospital, to the same day	3856
Of which number have died	1002

Source: Based on Cohen (7), p. 197.

of inoculation. An example comes from the study of another preventive approach published in 1994 (8).

In this case the question being addressed is whether immunizing older patients with flu vaccine at the time of an influenza epidemic is effective in reducing rates of hospitalization among senior citizens. The study uses data from subjects who are enrolled in a large health maintenance organization (HMO) in the Minneapolis–St. Paul area of Minnesota. The administrative health records of more than 25,000 people aged 65 and older who belong to the HMO form the basis for analysis. During the winter of 1991–1992 an epidemic of influenza occurred in the Minneapolis area. Prior to the outbreak, 58% of the older HMO enrollees had been recently immunized against influenza and 42% had not. The investigators examined the records to identify patients who had been hospitalized for various reasons, including pneumonia and influenza. They found a difference between those who had and those who had not received the flu vaccine. A rate of 7.1 hospitalizations per 1000 subjects is found for vaccinees, compared with a rate of 9.5 hospitalizations for every 1000 of those who had not been vaccinated. The comparison of these two rates indicates that, all other things being equal (assuming the groups are comparable in other risks that might lead to hospitalization), influenza vaccination is responsible for a 25% reduction in hospitalization for pneumonia and influenza.

That sounds reasonable. Immunization against influenza doesn't completely eliminate these hospitalizations, but it lessens them by a sizable margin. But the assumption "all other things being equal," requires examination. Was the risk of hospitalization (apart from the vaccine) similar for subjects who received vaccines compared with those who did not? Were the groups similar in age? Were they similar in general health status? Were they comparable with respect to chronic health problems that might predispose to hospitalization? If the only feature that differentiates the groups is the presence or absence of the flu vaccine, then we can feel that it is responsible for the reductions. But are we confident such is the case? To address this question the investigators collected information on a number of subject attributes that might predispose those subjects to hospitalization. A list of these is seen in Table 2-4.

The table shows that vaccinees and nonvaccinees are similar in age and in the distribution of males and females. But more revealing

TABLE 2-4

Characteristics of Study Subjects, According to Vaccination
Status, Minneapolis–St. Paul, 1991–1992

Characteristic	Vaccine	No Vaccine
Number of subjects	15,288	11,081
Average age (years)	72.0	72.5
Male sex (%)	45.2	41.8
Female sex (%)	54.8	58.2
Visits to physician in prior 12 months	14.3	8.5
Current medical problems:		
Coronary heart disease	15.5	8.9
Chronic lung disease	9.9	6.4
Diabetes	10.8	6.4
Pneumonia during previous 12 mo. (%)	4.1	2.5

Source: Based on Nichol (8).

differences emerge as we move down the table. Vaccinees visit
physicians more frequently, averaging over 14 visits in a 12-month
period, compared with 8.5 for nonvaccinees. Vacinees also have
more medical problems, including heart disease, lung disease, and
diabetes. More of them had pneumonia during the previous year.
The groups are not alike. The vaccinated group has poorer health,
more medical problems. Should we be surprised? Probably not.
Doctors are more likely to administer flu vaccine to patients who
have underlying problems such as heart or lung disease or diabetes. These patients are more vulnerable to influenza.

What does this lack of comparability between our groups
mean for our natural experiment on the efficacy of flu vaccine? If all
things are *not* equal, can we say the vaccine is beneficial? How
might results be altered if the vaccinees are less healthy from the
outset? Examine the difference in hospitalization rates again. The
more chronically ill vaccinees had a *lower* rate. Without vaccination,
the rate would likely have been *higher* than that of the comparison,
unvaccinated group. The 25% reduction in hospitalizations attributed to the flu vaccine is probably an underestimate of the vaccine's
value. Had the vaccinees not been immunized, their rate would
likely have been higher than that of the comparison group.

Subjects in this study who received vaccine are a *selected* group. They are not *representative*, or typical of 72-year-olds who reside in Minneapolis–St. Paul. They became part of the natural experiment because they had medical conditions that put them at greater risk from the flu and prompted their doctors to immunize them. That makes for good medical care. But it causes mischief in the medical experiment. If we really want to know whether flu-immunized older folks are less likely to be hospitalized than those who don't get the vaccine, the "playing field" should be level. The groups being compared should have an equal chance of experiencing the outcome (in this case, hospitalization) in the absence of the intervention (in this case, the flu vaccination).

In the present example, lack of comparable risk at the outset could have hidden a benefit of the vaccine. The vaccinated and nonvaccinated groups could have shown no difference in their hospitalization rates, not because the vaccine was ineffective, but because the benefit of vaccine was not large enough to overcome the greater burden of illness present among vaccinees *before* the experiment began. This problem is known as a *selection bias*. It is a major threat to the interpretation of medical research. The bias occurs whenever the allocation of subjects into groups is influenced by factors that are related to the outcome. In the flu vaccine case, sicker patients were chosen to receive the intervention because they were thought to be more likely to become seriously ill (and require hospitalization) if they were to contract influenza. In this instance, the benefits of the vaccine more than compensated for the unequal risk. But selection bias doesn't always operate in that direction.

A current treatment question of intense interest is whether giving estrogen replacement to postmenopausal women is beneficial. The practice of providing supplemental hormone when natural estrogen production declines in midlife was begun in earnest in the 1960s and was heavily promoted. Replacement estrogen alleviated unpleasant symptoms such as hot flashes, insomnia, and vaginal dryness associated with menopause. But because it was also observed that rates of heart disease in women rose following menopause it was hypothesized that hormone replacement therapy (HRT) might be beneficial in preventing heart attacks as well.

Indeed, a number of medical studies suggested such was the case. Using natural experiment data, it was found that women who took HRT after menopause had lower rates of dying from heart attack than women who did not. In some of the studies the difference was striking—reductions as much as 50%. The evidence for the benefit of HRT was seen in multiple studies. But there was a concern. As with the case of the influenza vaccine, there is a question of the comparability of women who use HRT and those who don't. Are all things equal in the comparison, save the use of estrogens by one set of women? Might there be differences between the groups that influence the outcome, heart disease?

Investigators from Pittsburgh approached this question by examining a group of premenopausal women for characteristics that were known to be related to the development of heart disease (9). These so-called risk factors include education, weight, alcohol intake, physical activity, smoking status, and blood pressure. Low education, excess weight, nondrinking, low physical activity, and cigarette smoking are all related to contracting heart disease. The researchers reevaluated this group of women periodically to track those who became postmenopausal and subsequently began HRT. Table 2-5 shows what they found.

Hormone replacement users have a different heart disease risk profile from nonusers. They are better educated, weigh less,

TABLE 2-5

Characteristics of Hormone Replacement Users and Nonusers in Pittsburgh, PA, 1983–1992

Characteristic	Users	Nonusers
Number of women	157	170
Education, at least some college (%)	81	63
Weight (in kilograms)	64.2	68.5
Alcohol intake (in grams per day)	9.7	7.5
Weekly physical activity (in kjoules*)	7160	5120
Current smoker (%)	29	34

*A measure of physical energy expenditure

Source: Based on Matthews (9).

drink a bit more alcohol, are more physically active, and are somewhat less likely to smoke. All these characteristics suggest that, before they even begin the treatment, individuals in the HRT group are less likely to develop coronary heart disease and subsequent heart attacks. They begin the experiment with an advantage. No level playing field here. This variant of selection bias, where individuals who receive intervention are predisposed to a more *favorable* outcome than the comparison group makes the interpretation of results difficult. Are favorable health outcomes caused by the HRT or by the lower inherent risk of heart disease among the women who choose treatment?[1]

Selection bias is a widespread and significant bugbear in the determination of the benefits of all sorts of preventive and therapeutic interventions. It means that while Mather, Boylston, and Franklin can be credited with using an innovative approach to evaluating efficacy, the challenge of deciding whether interventions like inoculation work is more formidable than first appears. Were the colonists who received inoculation at the same risk of dying from smallpox as those who developed disease "the natural way"? Could they have been better off financially, better nourished, healthier, and less likely to have perished from the disease without the intervention? We don't know. We will return to the problem of selection bias and the issue of hormone replacement therapy later.

The story of smallpox inoculation in the American colonies offers some important lessons. The case fatality comparisons between naturally occurring and inoculation-induced cases represent the first time data were collected and used to determine whether a public health intervention actually improved health. The data demonstrated that smallpox cases created by inoculation were far less likely to end in fatalities than cases that contracted the disease in "the common way." The conclusion was supported by repeated observations made on different populations in different places at different times.

Zabdiel Boylston proved resilient to the assaults of William Douglass and James Franklin. In 1723 he was invited to England to share his experiences with inoculation. While there, he lectured to

---

[1] Recent data from more rigorous experiments have revealed some detrimental effects of HRT on the heart and support the suspicion of slection bias. There will be more on the topic in Chapter 9.

the Royal College of Physicians and was elected to membership in the Royal Society. He also wrote and published "An Historical Account of the Smallpox Inoculated in New England," a monograph in which he gave details on his cases and compiled statistics on the new procedure. He returned to the colonies in 1726, where he settled back into practice and continued to promote inoculation.

Douglass continued to snipe at Boylston and Mather, though reluctantly he began to admit that inoculation had some promise as smallpox preventive:

> I heartily wish Success to this and all other Means designed to alleviate the Epidemic Distempers incident to Mankind; whether casually discovered, or ingeniously contrived by the Sons of Aesculapius: But rashness and head-strong irregular procedure I shall forever exclaim against, especially that detestable Wickedness of spreading Infection. (1, p. 71)

Science had beaten prejudice. But Douglass could never quite forgive the intrusion of the clergy and the lesser-trained Boylston in bringing inoculation to the fore of medical practice. He insisted that the procedure be restricted by the legislature and be performed by "abler hands, than Greek old Women, Madmen, and Fools" (1, p. 71).

Mather also withstood the controversy and returned to his flock. His remaining 7 years of life were arduous. His personal life was plagued by debt and family discord. His marital relations caused him constant distress, and his oldest son died at sea, the 12th of his children to perish. He continued his ministerial duties and his lifelong passion for writing, producing 39 titles during the last 2 years of his life. He also continued to dabble in science and medicine, and in 1724 he produced the first medical text written in the New World. The *Angel of Bethesda: An Essay upon the Common Maladies of Mankind* took its title from a legendary healing pool in the Holy Land. In the text, Mather rambled through the sources, symptoms, and solutions to a variety of illnesses, from toothaches to piles, including consumption, gout, measles, and of course, smallpox. It was a remarkable volume in its prescience, for in it he hinted at concepts of immunology and microbiology that were not to be "discovered" until many decades later. Mather had recognized the principle that underlies the success of inoculation, that individuals who contract an illness are protected from the disease thereafter. This is the basis for our present-day science of immunology, the science that has protected us against a multiplicity of diseases with a multiplicity of vaccines.

Mather had another notion as well—that smallpox "may be more of an animalculated business than we have been generally aware of." Cognizant of the early microscopic observations of the Dutchman, Antony van Leeuwenhoek, Mather had come to believe that "we walk through unseen Armies of numberless Living Things ready to seize and prey upon us." He hypothesized that these unseen swarms of minute animals could invade the body, multiply therein, and cause disease. He even suggested a specificity to these attacking microbes as "one Species of these Animals may offend in one Way, and another in another, and the various Parts may be variously offended: from whence may flow a Variety of Diseases" (10, pp. 87–90). Although arguably reminiscent of his "unseen world of demons," this theory had a somewhat better scientific basis. It would be 150 years before others would confirm that it was true.

Mather was close to several modern truths. But he lacked the scientific tools available to later generations. He was in the wrong century and the wrong profession. His substantial intelligence lacked an environment that could nurture his ideas. His history becomes that of a cranky dilettante rather than a celebrated scientist. His legacy comes from the foolish pronouncements on the invisible world of devils rather than his insights on microorganisms. His personality didn't help. Mather was pontifical, peevish, self-pitying, pedantic, petty, and provocative. But for all his faults he possessed a genuine humanitarian spirit. He even had the generosity to pass on hard-earned advice to sometime adversaries. Several years after Mather had been pilloried in the Franklin brothers' newspaper, he invited the younger Franklin to his home. At the conclusion of the visit, Mather was showing his guest out through a narrow passageway that had a low-lying ceiling beam. Franklin reports:

> We were all talking as I withdrew, he accompanying me behind, and I turning partly towards him, when he said hastily, "*Stoop, stoop!*" I did not understand him till I felt my head hit against the beam. He was a man that never missed any occasion of giving instruction, and upon this he said to me: "*You are young, and you have the world before you; STOOP as you go through it, and you will miss many hard thumps.*" (3, p. 383)

It was good advice for a disordered time.

REFERENCES

1. Blake JB. *Public Health in the Town of Boston 1630–1822.* Cambridge, MA: Harvard University Press; 1959.
2. Thacher J. *American Medical Biography, or Memoirs of Eminent Physicians Who Have Flourished in America.* New York: Milford House; 1967.
3. Silverman K. *The Life and Times of Cotton Mather.* New York: Welcome Rain Publishers; 1984.
4. Hopkins DR. *Princes and Peasants: Smallpox in History.* Chicago: The University of Chicago Press; 1983.
5. Mather C. *Diary of Cotton Mather.* New York: F. Ungar Pub Co; 1957.
6. Fitz RH. Zabdiel Boylston, inoculator, and the epidemic of smallpox in Boston in 1721. *Bulletin of the Johns Hopkins Hospital.* 1911:22; 315–327.
7. Cohen IB. *Benjamin Franklin.* Indianapolis: Bobbs-Merrill Co Inc; 1953.
8. Nichol KL, Margolis KL, Wuorenma J, Von Sternberg T. The efficacy and cost effectiveness of vaccination against influenza among elderly persons living in the community. *N Engl J Med.* 1994; 331:778–784.
9. Matthews KA, Kuller LH, Wing RR, Meilahn EN, Plantinga P. Prior to use of estrogen replacement therapy, are users healthier than nonusers? *Am J Epidemiol.* 1996; 143:971–978.
10. Beall OT, Jr. , Shryock RH. *Cotton Mather: First Significant Figure in American Medicine.* Baltimore: Johns Hopkins Press; 1954.

CHAPTER 3

Noddle's Island Experiment: Benjamin Waterhouse and Vaccination

Noddle's Island can no longer be found on the map of Massachusetts—at least not on any recent map. Once the largest of Boston's harbor islands, its marshy acreage lay just a half-mile across the water from the town's busiest wharf. Now, it lies beneath tons of brick and concrete—the condominiums, shops, and markets of East Boston—and is neighbor to the frenetic activity of Logan International Airport. Two hundred years ago, Noddle's Island was considerably less peopled and a great deal more isolated. In fact, it was because of its isolation, outside the town limits of Boston, that Noddle's was selected for its historic role. In the late autumn of 1802 the island became the site of America's first planned public health experiment.

The experiment took place on November 9, when 13 boys from the town were ferried to the island, established in a small wooden building that had been erected for the specific occasion, and inoculated with smallpox. The inoculation procedure was, of course, by this time no longer novel. The event that preceded it was.

Plans for the experiment had begun almost 6 months earlier, when Dr. Benjamin Waterhouse, a local physician, had petitioned the Board of Health for permission to test an exciting new technique for preventing smallpox. The principle behind the new procedure was similar to that of inoculation. A subject's skin was abraded with a sharp implement, then inoculated with a small amount of infectious virus. In this instance, however, the agent was not the smallpox virus but a country cousin, a virus that produced a pox-like disease among cows.

The disease was known as kine-pox or cowpox. It was an ailment that had been known for centuries in rural areas of England, where dairy maids who milked infected cows developed pustules on their hands and wrists. Among the country folk it was widely believed that an individual who had experienced cowpox was protected from the ravages of smallpox. This theory, while broadly accepted in rural farming communities, had escaped the serious attention of members of the medical profession, who regarded it at best a "curiosity." Then, in the last decade of the 18th century, a country doctor from Gloucestershire became intrigued with the observation and decided it merited serious evaluation.

Edward Jenner was born in Berkeley, England, in 1749. He had listened to stories of the marvelous powers of kine-pox from his earliest years. Jenner passed his preliminary medical training in the apprenticeship tradition with Mr. Ludlow, a surgeon from Chipping Sodbury. He then went to London to study with the well-known English surgeon, John Hunter. Hunter and Jenner became close friends, sharing interests not only in medicine but in the natural sciences. When Jenner returned to his native Berkeley to set up practice in 1773, he maintained a lively correspondence with Hunter. Subjects ranged from the core body temperature of hibernating hedgehogs to the composition of whale's milk to determining the sex of eels. In fact, Jenner, whose name is now synonymous with smallpox vaccination, achieved his earliest scientific distinction and election to the Royal Society not for the landmark contribution to preventative medicine but for his observations on the nesting behavior of cuckoos.

Kine-pox fascinated Jenner. Recalling the anecdotes of the protective benefits of cowpox from his youth, he began collecting stories, case histories that supported his developing hypothesis that cowpox protected from smallpox.

> – Sarah Portlock, of this place, was infected with the cowpox when a servant at a farmer's in the neighbourhood, twenty-seven years ago.
> In the year 1792, conceiving herself, from this circumstance, secure from the infection of the smallpox, she nursed one of her own children who had accidentally caught the disease, but no indisposition ensued. During the

time she remained in the infected room, variolous matter was inserted into both her arms, but without any further effect than in the preceding case.

– Mrs. H –, a respectable gentlewoman of this town had the cow-pox when very young. She received the infection in rather an uncommon manner: it was given by means of her handling some of the same utensils which were in use among the servants of the family, who had the disease from milking infected cows. Her hands had many of the cow-pox sores upon them, and they were communicated to her nose, which became inflamed and very much swollen. Soon after this event Mrs. H – was exposed to the contagion of the smallpox, where it was scarcely possible for her to have escaped, had she been susceptible of it, as she regularly attended a relative who had the disease in so violent a degree that it proved fatal to him. (1)

Two lines of evidence emerged to support the belief that cow-pox was protective. The first was based on the finding that individuals who had a history of contracting cowpox years before did not come down with smallpox even when subjected to intensive exposure to naturally occurring disease in later years. They could eat and sleep in the same room as smallpox victims, nurse them, attend them constantly, without ill effects.

The second evidence was even stronger. Those experienced with cowpox would not react to inoculation. When challenged with a dose of infectious matter from an active smallpox patient in the standard procedure introduced by Boylston, they showed no response. No pustules, no swollen glands, not even a mild case of smallpox. At most, they would display a slight redness and swelling at the sight of the incision and implantation.

Case reports or histories provide valuable bits of evidence—useful first steps toward proving medical hypotheses. But they are not sufficient in themselves. Jenner's collection of case histories emboldened him to take on the next necessary step, the role of experimenter. He began by inoculating patients who had a history of prior cowpox infection and observing their reactions:

– John Phillips, a tradesman of this town, had the cow-pox at so early a period as nine years of age. At the age of sixty-two I inoculated him, and was very careful in selecting matter in its most active state. It was taken from the arm of a boy just before the commencement of the eruptive fever, and instantly inserted. It very speedily produced a sting-like feel in the part. An efflorescence appeared, which on the fourth day was rather extensive, and some degree of pain and stiffness were felt about the shoulder; but on the fifth day these symptoms began to disappear, and in a day or two after went entirely off, without producing any effect on the system.

In the year 1778 the smallpox prevailed very much at Berkeley, and Mrs. H –, not feeling perfectly satisfied respecting her safety (no indisposition having followed her exposure to the smallpox), I inoculated her with active variolous matter. The same appearance followed as in the preceding cases—an efflorescence on the arm without any effect on the constitution. (1)

The absence of more than mild local reactions to his inoculations convinced Jenner that cowpox was protective. He took another step. In May 1796, he was attending Sarah Nelmes, a local dairy maid, who had become infected with cowpox. Nelmes had developed a large pustule on her hand at the spot where she had been previously scratched by a thorn. Jenner extracted some pus from the lesion and, on May 14, inserted it into the arm of a healthy 8-year-old boy "by means of two superficial incisions, barely penetrating cutis, each about half an inch long." (see Figure 3-1) It was

FIGURE 3-1

Edward Jenner Performs the First Vaccination

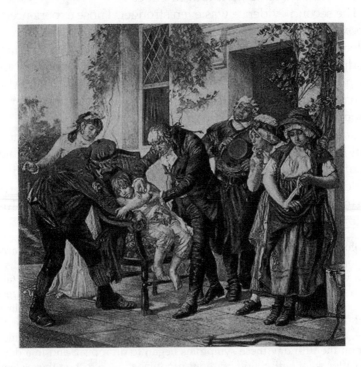

Source: From a photogravure by Melingue, National Library of Medicine.

a simple statement to describe one of the most singular events in public health history. The boy, James Phipps, experienced a mild reaction to this first vaccination.*

> On the 7th day he complained of uneasiness in the axilla (armpit), and on the 9th he became a little chilly, lost his appetite, and had a slight headache. During the whole of this day he was perceptively indisposed and spent the night with some degree of restlessness, but on the day following he was perfectly well (1).

Jenner noted that the lesion induced by vaccination was similar in appearance and healed in much the same way as incisions inoculated with actual smallpox virus.

Then Jenner performed the real test. Six weeks after the vaccination, he obtained infectious material from the pustule of a smallpox patient and inoculated it onto both of James's arms. Jenner watched his subject carefully over the next two weeks. The incisions became slightly red and tender but there were no pustules, no headache and fever, no systemic signs of illness—*no smallpox*. Several months later, he again inoculated James with material obtained from an active smallpox patient "but no sensible effect was produced on the constitution"(1).

Jenner reported his stunning results in June 1798, in a pamphlet entitled *An Inquiry Into the Causes and Effects of Variolae Vaccinae, a Disease Discovered in Some of the Western Counties of England, Particularly Gloucestershire, and Known by the Name of Cowpox*. It seemed, a later commentator would write, "as if an angel's trumpet had sounded over the earth" (2, p. 79). Three years later Jenner was to make a bold prediction about the discovery: "It now becomes too manifest to admit of controversy, that the

---

* The term *vaccination* derives from the Latin *vaca*, or cow, for obvious reasons. From here on the terminology is a bit tricky. We've been speaking for two chapters now about *inoculation*. As used, the term referred to the specific act of engrafting or infecting individuals with *variola*, the virus that causes smallpox, to protect them from getting the disease. Now Jenner uses the same technique of introducing a virus into an abrasion on the skin. But he uses a slightly different virus, the cowpox virus, and calls the procedure *vaccination*. Today we use the terms inoculation and vaccination almost interchangeably. They have both become generic terms to describe a variety of protective, immunizing agents. For example, we inoculate or vaccinate against polio, influenza, and diphtheria. For purposes of our present discussion, however, the terms will be used in their original, limited meanings: *inoculation* referring only to implanting the *variola* virus, *vaccination* to using cowpox.

annihilation of the Small Pox, the most dreadful scourge of the human species, must be the final result of this practice"(3).

In America, the news reached Benjamin Waterhouse that following winter. Waterhouse was arguably the best-educated medical man the new republic could boast. He was born in Newport, Rhode Island, in 1754, and raised as a Quaker—a peaceable tradition that was not entirely in harmony with his temperament. His teenage years were spent in the usual medical apprenticeships with local physicians. On the eve of the Revolution, in 1775, he was sent to London to enhance his education. Over the next 6 years he studied with one of England's most distinguished physicians, Dr. John Fothergill, took classes in Edinburgh and Leyden, and rubbed elbows with such scientific luminaries as John Hunter, William Cullen, Joseph Priestly, and Benjamin Franklin. He shared lodgings with long-time friend and painter Gilbert Stuart and served as model for a Stuart portrait (see Figure 3-2).

FIGURE 3-2

Benjamin Waterhouse

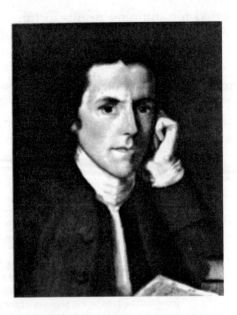

Source: From a painting by Stuart, National Library of Medicine.

Waterhouse returned to America with medical credentials that were difficult to equal, and ambitions to match. He was intent on transforming backwater American medicine to the sophisticated science he had experienced in Europe. Soon after his return, he was appointed as the first professor of Theory and Practice of Physic (one of only 3) at the nascent school of medicine at Harvard. Like many educated men of his time, his interests were broad. He lectured on natural history as well as medicine, and he established a botanical garden in Cambridge. Among his early contributions at Harvard was his "Cautions to Young Persons Concerning Health," a lecture he gave with some regularity, admonishing the students on the ruinous effects of smoking cigars and the dangers of demon rum. Waterhouse proclaimed that the Harvard student of the day was in stagnation and decline, asserting that "six times as much ardent spirits were expended here [in Cambridge] annually as in days of our fathers. Unruly wine and ardent spirits have supplanted sober cider" (4, p. 276).

Waterhouse first learned of vaccination from an English acquaintance who, in November 1798, wrote of the exciting discovery that had just been reported by Jenner. A copy of Jenner's treatise followed the letter. Waterhouse was impressed. He reported the discovery in the local paper, the *Columbian Sentinel*, and assiduously followed the reports from England on the growing use of vaccination. He and his colleagues in America were impatient to try the new preventative. Finally, in July 1800, he obtained a small amount of vaccine from England. His first subject, like that of Zabdiel Boylston, was his own son. Five-year-old Daniel became the first American to receive cowpox. Then 3 more of Waterhouse's children and 3 servants were vaccinated. Waterhouse waited several weeks for the vaccination to take effect. He then persuaded Dr. William Aspinwall, who owned and operated a hospital in Brookline dedicated to smallpox inoculation, to inoculate his 7 subjects. None of the cowpox vaccinees developed smallpox. Energized by the success of his experiment, Waterhouse began to publicize his ability to perform the procedure. By the end of August he had vaccinated 50 people.

The observations that led to both inoculation and vaccination were similar, that individuals who had recovered from smallpox infection, whether natural or artificially induced, or infection with cowpox were resistant to future attacks from the *variola* (smallpox) virus.

Jenner and Waterhouse, as well as Mather and Boylston before them, had identified, though not articulated, the basic concept of the immune response. They discovered the body's system of defense against a world of external threats. This immune response is triggered whenever unfamiliar, foreign protein penetrates our outer defenses: the skin or respiratory or intestinal membranes. Cells of the immune system mobilize to track down these invaders and a cascade of events is initiated during which the body attempts not only to repel the interlopers but to construct a defense against similar attacks in the future. Activated cells from the blood and adjacent tissues attempt to engulf and destroy invading organisms. This activity takes considerable effort and sometimes becomes a literal life and death struggle. By the time the system recognizes the invasion, the organisms have already gained a foothold. They have multiplied in lymph nodes close to the point of entry and begun to spread to other parts of the body. It takes some time to resolve the problem. The 3 to 4 weeks it takes for smallpox to run its course, from the time of infection to the healing of the last scab that was described earlier, is a case in point.

At the same time that this contest is going on, immune responsive cells are identifying and cataloging the unique structure of the *antigen* (foreign protein) that has been introduced. A memory bank is created so that the next time the antigen is encountered, the body can immediately respond to ward off the infection before it takes hold. Certain preprogrammed cells (*B cells*) multiply and secrete antibodies that coat the offending virus or bacterium. Other cells (*T cells*) attack the antigen directly. The critical feature is the specificity of the response. The immune system only recognizes and reacts to antigens that have been seen before. With inoculation, it is easy to see how the process works since inoculation actually produces a case of smallpox. Once patients recover, they are primed to reject subsequent invasions by the virus. The cowpox virus differs from smallpox only slightly and its structure is similar enough to fool the immune system. A system that has experienced cowpox responds quickly and effectively to ward off infection by the more dangerous smallpox virus.

Once the public became aware of the success of Waterhouse's experiments, both patients and other physicians clamored to obtain the "vaccine." Here, Waterhouse made a mistake that was to haunt him for the rest of his days. Under the pretence of keeping the vaccine out of the hands of the inexperienced and incompetent, he refused to share his vaccine widely. This withholding was viewed by many as an attempt by Waterhouse to gain a monopoly and fatten his personal pocketbook rather than as protection of the public health. Indeed, the selected physicians with whom he did share his treasure had to agree to send 25% of the profits they received from administering the vaccine to Waterhouse. Growing public pressure and competing alternative sources ultimately forced him to abandon his monopolistic approach and broadened distribution of the vaccine. But residual resentment smoldered for many years thereafter.

By the spring of 1802 considerable enthusiasm for vaccination had developed among the physicians and citizens of Boston. But there were still skeptics and detractors. Many, not trusting the new technique, continued to subject themselves to the more dangerous practice of inoculation and continued to patronize smallpox inoculation hospitals such as Aspinwall's. Waterhouse decided it was time for a public demonstration of the benefits of vaccination. He petitioned the Board of Health for permission to conduct a public experiment. The board was at first reluctant but finally, after consulting a number of the town's leading physicians, agreed that the idea had merit. There were obstacles, however. Waterhouse's plan required that a group of subjects who had been vaccinated with cowpox would be challenged with smallpox inoculation to prove the protective power of the vaccine. But the town meeting refused to grant permission "on the grounds that it would alarm the country and injure the trade of the town"(5). Much debate ensued. Finally it was agreed that the Board of Health could carry on the experiment but it would have to conduct the inoculation challenge outside of town. That decision led to the creation of the small-frame building on Noddle's Island.

The experiment was begun on August 16. Nineteen of the town's children, who had been volunteered by their parents, were assembled at the health office and, under the watchful eye of Boston's most respected physicians, vaccinated with cowpox. By the time the logistics and location for the challenge could be arranged it was November. On the 9th of the month, 12 of the boys plus another young man who had been given cowpox earlier were reassembled at the temporary hospital on Noddle's Island. There, each was inoculated with freshly gathered "matter" from the pustules of an active smallpox patient. In addition, the 2 sons of Christopher Clark of Hinchmen Lane, young men who had not experienced either smallpox or cowpox, were also inoculated. All the boys were closely observed over the next 2 weeks. The arms of the Clark boys became inflamed. They developed fevers and broke out in pustules, about 500 on one child and 150 on the other. The other 13 children were "totally unaffected" (5). On November 21, material from the pustules of the Clarks was gathered and the 13 were reinoculated. Again they remained well. As a final proof, Waterhouse insisted that all the children remain together for the duration of the experiment, in the same house, in the same room, and often in the same beds. They still remained well.

Ten of the town's doctors in addition to Waterhouse visited the hospital at Noddle's periodically to observe the progress of the experiment. In mid-December they all signed a statement attesting to the efficacy of the cowpox vaccine. It read:

> Each of the children was examined by the subscribers, who were individually convinced from the inspection of their arms, their perfect state of health, and exemption from every kind of eruption on their bodies, that the cowpox prevented their taking the smallpox, and they do therefore consider the result of the experiment as satisfactory evidence that the cowpox is a complete security against the smallpox. (5)

It was an extraordinary event in the history of American medical science. Benjamin Waterhouse had designed and carried out an experiment on human subjects. He had applied his preventive vaccine to a group of young boys and then deliberately challenged them with smallpox to see if the vaccination worked. But this was not the most remarkable part. Jenner had also challenged his vaccinees with smallpox some years earlier. What Waterhouse added was the 2 untreated comparison subjects. Children who had no prior exposure to either cowpox or smallpox were included with his experimental innoculees. This step adds a significant level of sophistication to the experiment.

Untreated comparison subjects help us sort out *alternative explanations* for our experimental results. Waterhouse recognized that there were several possible interpretations for the outcome of his experiment. When subjects who receive cowpox vaccine show no reaction to their subsequent challenge with the smallpox virus, no pustules and no fever, the obvious interpretation is that the cowpox protects against smallpox. But there is another possibility. Suppose that the agent used for the smallpox challenge had lost its potency. Suppose that the "smallpox matter" used had been improperly collected, or subjected to excessive heat and rendered inactive. Experience with inoculation programs had shown that, if improperly handled, smallpox inoculation material could lose its viability. Under such circumstances, Waterhouse's vaccinated subjects would have failed to demonstrate response to inoculation, not because the vaccine protected them but because the challenge virus was impotent. When untreated comparison subjects are included in the experiment, and they develop disease typical of inoculation smallpox, the competing explanation for the findings is eliminated. The challenge dose is active, so the vaccine must be protective.

Inclusion of an untreated comparison group in an experiment adds greatly to its explanatory power. Consider another, more recent immunization example—another disease that has pestered people for as long as smallpox, albeit in a less serious manner. Disdainfully known as "the common cold," upper respiratory tract infections (URIs) cause more loss of work than loss of life, more minor misery than mortality. Nonetheless, an effective preventive to this perennial problem would be of an unquestioned benefit.

Colds, like smallpox, are caused by a virus, or rather, a variety of them—over 100 different types of *rhinovirus* (*rhino* referring to nose) have been associated with the symptoms of runny nose, congestion, cough, sore throat, and aches that are the hallmark of the common cold. And that becomes part of the problem in trying to develop a preventive agent. These multiple viruses all have slightly different antigenic configurations. Unlike the convenient similarity between cowpox and smallpox viruses, the subgroups of rhinovirus aren't enough alike that immunity against one provides protection against another. Each requires a specific immune response from the body. This complexity makes developing effective immunizing agents against colds a formidable challenge.

Back in the 1920s and 1930s, we knew much less about the viral nature of URIs than we do today. In part, this ignorance was bliss, as demonstrated by the considerable enthusiasm for vaccines made from inactivated bacterial components that were promoted as preventatives for the common cold.* A notable experiment to evaluate the efficacy of one of these vaccines was conducted in the "cold friendly" climate of Minneapolis, Minnesota. (6) There, researchers at the University of Minnesota, following the example set by Waterhouse 135 years earlier, recruited a group of young volunteers for an experiment. In this case, the subjects were students at the university. All were healthy young men and women save for one characteristic: each was selected for study because of a particular "susceptibility" to colds.

At the time of enrollment, every student was examined. A thorough history was obtained, which documented the frequency and severity of colds experienced in the previous year and the number of days lost from school as a result of the infections. Subjects were then injected with a vaccine made from 5 inactivated bacteria twice each week for 3 weeks, then every 2 weeks throughout the school year. Students were instructed to report any symptoms of a cold to staff at the health service. Monthly reports were obtained from each subject, and the physicians who cared for them kept careful notes on the severity and symptoms of each cold they observed.

All this activity seems a great deal of effort. But it was worth it. After 2 years of study, the results were dramatic. For the 272 students who completed the experiment, the rate of colds fell from an average of 5.9 per year in the 12 months before the experiment to an average of only 1.6 per year while the vaccine program was ongoing. That is a reduction of 73%. It is easy to conclude that the vaccine is beneficial.

But the Minnesota investigators took another page from Waterhouse's text. They included comparison subjects. At the very start of the experiment, the student volunteers were split into 2 groups. The first, the 272 just described, was given the active bacterial vaccine. But a second group, of equal size, became the control group. They received injections on the same schedule as the experimental group but with saltwater instead of vaccine. All the students

---

* By this time, "vaccine" had been appropriated to mean any immunizing agent against disease and was not restricted to immunizations utilizing cowpox.

were under the impression that they were receiving the active immunization.

When the results for the control group were tabulated, they were also remarkable, as Table 3-1 shows: a 63% reduction in colds, from an average of 5.6 the previous year to 2.1 in the study year. These findings are very close to those for the active vaccine recipients. The average number of days lost from school was also similar. It is an unexpected result, one that forces a revision in our earlier conclusions about the efficacy of the cold vaccine. An apparent victory for preventive medicine has been undone by the use of the comparison group.

But this is good, not unhappy news. The goal of an experiment is, after all, to learn the truth. Does the cold vaccine prevent URIs? Prior to this experiment and several like it, cold vaccines had come into widespread and uncritical use. Hundreds of thousands of persons throughout the country had been jabbed with these vaccines in hopes of warding off URIs. In addition to raising thousands of false expectations, the practice resulted in many unnecessary office visits, wasted time and money, and more than one or two sore arms. The information gained from the controlled experiment sets this aright.*

TABLE 3-1

Average Number of Colds per Year and Days Lost from School for Cold Vaccine Subjects and Saltwater Comparison Group

Average Number of Colds per Year	Cold Vaccine ($n = 272$)	Saltwater ($n = 276$)
Previous year	5.9	5.6
Study year	1.6	2.1
Average days lost from school during study year	1.1	1.0

Source: Based on Diehl et al. (6).

---

* Additional evidence that casts doubt on the efficacy of this vaccine is biological rather than methodological. The vaccine was composed of a number of inactivated strains of bacteria. Since we now appreciate that colds are brought on by rhinoviruses, not bacteria, there is no immunologic basis to believe that bacterial immunizing agents would be successful.

But how do we explain such results? Why would the rate of colds decline so precipitously in both the experimental and comparison groups? There are other explanations for the reduction in colds from the one year to the next. To begin with, the severity of cold seasons fluctuates from year to year. During some winters, respiratory diseases are particularly abundant—everyone is suffering from repeated colds. In other years, there are not so many URIs. It is a matter of *natural variation* in the occurrence of disease. It could well be that the winter before the experiment took place, the benchmark year, happened to be a particularly bad one for colds. Many people were sick. The next season, during the experiment, there were fewer respiratory viruses in the community. The reduction in colds experienced by the subjects reflects year-to-year variation in illnesses in the community, not the value of the vaccine.

It is also likely that there were differences in the way that colds were measured before the experiment began and during the course of the program. The "before" number was based on self-reports from the students. Each subject was the arbiter for the prior year's frequency and severity of colds and relied on memory of the events of the past 12 months. This measure is not a very trustworthy one. People have a tendency to compress events into shorter time frames than actually occur and to "enhance" the number of past events to meet the requirements of the study. After all, subjects knew they were being selected for their susceptibility to colds. One needed to report a convincing number of episodes to qualify for the study and be eligible for the vaccine.

On the other hand, the postvaccine colds were carefully recorded. Students were required to report their afflictions to the health center and have physicians verify their complaints. Each cold had to pass muster before it was tallied in the results. With such strict criteria for postvaccine colds, it's not surprising that the average number per individual fell.

There is another aspect to this "susceptibility" business in addition to the tendency of our memories to compress events and embellish the numbers to meet investigator's desires. As has been noted, the number of colds anyone experiences varies from year to year. In a good winter you may escape entirely; in a bad year, it may seem that one cold follows on the heels of another. The numbers are seldom consistent from year to year. They go up and down.

And because of this natural variability, an interesting phenomenon occurs when you select a group of people because they have very high (or low) values of an attribute like colds. It happens frequently in medical studies. Subjects are chosen for study particularly because they have too much or too little of something: blood pressure that is too high, red blood cells that are too few, cholesterol that is elevated, reduced bone density, or an excessive number of colds. They become part of the study and are treated—with a drug to lower blood pressure or cholesterol, or a medication to raise the red blood cells or bone density. They are then remeasured.

It turns out that subsequent measurements—those taken after subjects are admitted into the study—are likely to be less extreme (more toward normal) than the numbers that earned them entry in the first place. It has nothing to do with whether the treatment works. It is a statistical phenomenon known as *regression to the mean*, and its implications for medical research are profound. If these subjects, on average, are likely to have reduced blood pressures or higher bone density or fewer colds regardless of what therapeutic interventions are made, the risk of falsely attributing success to the treatment is obvious. But the truth is, the measurements improved not because of the treatment but because subjects' repeated measurements were, as expected, less extreme than on initial evaluation.

Having a comparison group travel alongside intervention subjects—people who are measured at the same time using the same criteria—helps us account for alternative explanations posed by natural variation in disease, measurement differences, and regression to the mean. Controls help us avoid drawing the wrong conclusion about the efficacy of a blood pressure medication or cold vaccine. We will see additional examples of ways that comparison groups help us deal with competing explanations later in the book.

The success of the Noddle's Island experiment bolstered an already favorable disposition toward vaccination among doctors and the public. The new preventive practice was accepted with surprising rapidity. Even before the success of the Waterhouse experiment was widely known, vaccination had spread up and down the eastern seaboard and as far west as Mississippi, Kentucky, and Ohio. It captured the attention of President Thomas Jefferson, who became a strong advocate after Waterhouse sent him some vaccine. Jefferson donated vaccine to several southern states as well as to several Native American tribes. Even early skeptics such as William Aspinwall, who had inoculated Waterhouse's 4 children with smallpox after they had received the cowpox, admitted that vaccination had advantages over inoculation. The admission was grudgingly given, as it was noted that abandoning the old procedure for the new would cost him dearly.

Nevertheless, bumps in the road remained. Public interest in preventing smallpox waned when there was no imminent threat of the disease. A vaccination institute founded in Boston shortly after the Noddle's Island experiment enjoyed immediate initial success. Almost 70 people were provided free vaccine in the first 2 months of operation. But within a year the public had become complacent, and the institute closed. There were also issues with the vaccine itself. Reports of smallpox cases occurring among people who were said to be immunized raised concerns about the quality of the cowpox vaccine in use. Indeed, there was evidence that not all the vaccine retained its immunizing potency, and there were clear instances of "spurious" vaccines in use. Because no standards for acquiring and handling the cowpox material existed, contamination occurred. An outbreak of smallpox following vaccination in Marblehead, Massachusetts, was attributed to unintended introduction of active smallpox virus. Occasionally, extensive inflammation developed at the site of vaccination and spread to other parts of the body. Though unexplained at the time, such episodes appear to be instances of contamination with pathogenic (disease-causing) bacteria. There were also concerns about the longevity of immunity conferred by the cowpox. Waterhouse staunchly defended the permanency of his product and rechallenged his own children with smallpox to prove they were still protected (7, pp. 182–183).

Some temporary setbacks not withstanding, vaccination marked the beginning of the end for smallpox, the "annihilation…of the most dreadful scourge of the human species," as Jenner had predicted. Though accurate data are difficult to come by, it was estimated that the rate of smallpox deaths in Massachusetts fell from 170 per million each year during the mid-1800s to 8 per million by the end of the century (2, p. 287). Epidemics did continue to occur sporadically throughout the century. This was particularly true in larger cities, where substantial numbers of unimmunized, often immigrant groups resided. Antivaccination factions added to the problem. These surfaced periodically in response to perceptions of abridged personal rights or reports of untoward reactions to vaccine. In addition, public health laws requiring vaccination were inconsistently implemented and enforced. Though legislation requiring vaccination of Massachusetts's children prior to school entry was enacted in 1855, the law was only rigorously enforced when new outbreaks of the disease were on the doorstep, as in 1870. California passed, and then repealed, a childhood immunization law, only to see the proportion of smallpox cases in children less than 15 years of age jump after the law was undone. As late as the 1930s, four states had passed laws *against* compulsory vaccination, an unwise decision that only further documented the value of vaccination. Figure 3-3 compares rates of smallpox by states

FIGURE 3-3

The Effect of Vaccination Laws on the Incidence of Smallpox in Various States

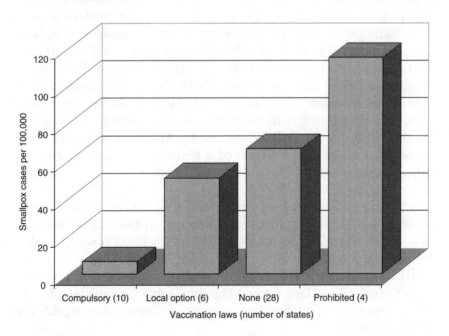

Source: Based on Woodward & Feemster (8, pp. 317–318).

according to the status of the state's smallpox vaccination laws and shows the value of the requirements (8).

After 1927, serious epidemics of smallpox were virtually eliminated from the United States. Several small outbreaks occurred in the 1940s, the result of importations of the disease from outside the country. The last of these was in 1949, when 8 cases and one death were reported from Texas, presumably after an infected individual crossed the border from Mexico. Following several decades of total absence of disease, vaccination programs were suspended in 1971. The adverse effects of the vaccine itself (while small) were causing more problems than "the most dreadful scourge of the human species."

The success of vaccination around the globe paralleled that in the United States. Several European countries made vaccination of infants compulsory early in the 19th century: Bavaria in 1807, Denmark in 1810, Norway in 1811, and Sweden in 1816. Periodic outbreaks of smallpox activity occurred after 1820, but were far less severe than before the introduction of vaccine. During these continuing epidemics, it was observed that cases occurred in previously vaccinated adults. While the individuals experienced a lower case-fatality rate than those who were unimmunized, it became clear that immunity was not as long-lived as Jenner and Waterhouse had hoped. Revaccination programs were developed. Following a large epidemic in Europe in the early 1870s, several German states introduced mandatory childhood vaccination in the second year of life, with revaccination in the 12th year. Comparing the smallpox mortality figures for Prussia and nearby Austria, where conditions were similar save the absence of a revaccination law in Austria, suggests substantial benefit to the smallpox vaccination law (see Table 3-2) (9, p. 273).

Ridding the entire globe of smallpox was a considerably more ambitious undertaking than eradication from the United States. It was a truly historic moment in public health when a hospital cook in the small town of Merka, Somalia, in East Africa, named Ali Maow Maalin, became the last known case of naturally occurring smallpox. Two years later, in December 1979, the Global Commission for the Certification of Smallpox Eradication proclaimed the world was smallpox-free.

TABLE 3 - 2

Average Number of Smallpox Deaths per Million Population for 3-Year Intervals Before and After Compulsory Vaccination and Revaccination Law of 1874 in Bavaria (Law Enacted) and Austria (no Revaccination Law)

Years	Bavaria	Austria
1866–1868	413	407
1869–1871	934	350
1872–1874	1025	2228
Revaccination Law Enacted		
1875–1877	23	512
1878–1880	15	613
1881–1883	31	783

Source: Based on Fenner (9).

Professional squabbles between Waterhouse and his colleagues grew despite the Noddle's Island success. Though Waterhouse insisted that all his actions related to the introduction of vaccination were for the public's welfare, his colleagues were unconvinced. They perceived pecuniary self-interest and were unable to forgive his early efforts to monopolize the vaccine and profit from the 25% charge he levied whenever he shared the precious product. Waterhouse defended himself in the popular press, claiming he only desired to prevent the inexperienced and incompetent from laying hands on the vaccine. He railed against the Medical Society for failing to support his efforts to "extend [the] power of illumination...of this new inoculation" (7, p. 56). The medical society replied, again suggesting that profit rather than professionalism were Waterhouse's principal concern. The debate became contentious, with heated exchanges in the popular press. The epistolary battle climaxed in 1806, with the Medical Society appearing to gain the last word.

He [Waterhouse] talks of the dignity of moderation, who has exhausted our language of abusive terms; he talks of personality, who has loaded with opprobrious epithets a most respectable physician; he declaims on the nicety of moral character, who has publicly violated the ninth commandment; he pretends to value himself for his "cardinal point of veracity," who before the world, has been proved guilty of repeated falsehoods. (7, pp. 58–59)

Waterhouse's reputation never did recover. He stayed at odds with his colleagues for the remainder of his life. In 1807. his friend, Thomas Jefferson, gave him a political post as physician to the marine hospital in Charlestown, Massachusetts. He lost it two years later when Jefferson left office. Waterhouse's fortunes at Harvard also declined. In 1809 he was dismissed from his post as "keeper of the mineralogical cabinet," and 3 years later the college removed him from his professorship. Not a spirit or an ego to be easily deflated, he continued his intellectual pursuits, reading broadly and writing prolifically. He reappeared in the public press from time to time to proselytize for causes in which he believed. At the age of 85, he published a commentary on the "great need for improvements as regards treatment of our horses and other beasts of labor" and 2 months later "condemned the carelessness which led to the frequent fires of Boston" (10, p. 363). He died in Cambridge in 1846 at the age of 92, still convinced of his value as "America's Jenner." His final diary entry, made at the age of 91, notes "some very useful things would probably never have existed or been postponed to a late and chilling distance of time, but for my exertions. I cut the claws and wings of smallpox....I am not, I hope, a boaster, but I have done my part" (10, p. 357).

The success enjoyed by smallpox vaccination was not shared by the research method that was introduced on Noddle's Island. The model—a closely observed and well-documented experiment in which one group of human subjects is administered a treatment and another group is left as an untreated comparison—has become a mainstay of present-day medical and public health research. The design that Waterhouse and the Board of Health introduced is now known as a *controlled clinical trial*. It is used to evaluate an array of public health and medical interventions that range from other immunizing agents (as we saw with the cold vaccine example) to drugs for lowering blood pressure and cholesterol, to surgical procedures such as coronary artery bypass, to drug addiction treatment programs, and health insurance programs. It is a powerful tool, which we will meet again in later chapters. But this bit of early 19th century research brilliance proved an unsustained moment of illumination. The approach did not take hold. It was not to be seen again until well over another century had passed.

One can only speculate why this was so. We have seen that much controversy existed in the early 19th century about the origins, nature, and spread of disease. Smallpox was one of the few diseases that was widely acknowledged to be specific, even if its precise cause was not known. The fortuitous discoveries of inoculation and, subsequently, vaccination, made its situation unique. Anecdotal evidence strongly suggested that cowpox protected against smallpox. Repeated stories told of those who had experienced the cowpox and were unaffected by a subsequent smallpox inoculation. These pointed directly to an obvious experiment: vaccinate with cowpox, then deliberately challenge with smallpox. The inclusion of the healthy, unvaccinated controls was prompted by the justified fear that the smallpox material might be impotent. Skeptics could discredit results by proposing the alternative explanation for the apparent efficacy of the vaccine—that is, that the challenge was invalid. These were special circumstances focused specifically on the smallpox problem. It alone came with a clear method for producing disease as well as a method for protection. No one saw the broader potential of the strategy. No one recognized that the controlled experiment might be used to test many other health interventions. Not one of the physicians who oversaw the affair at Noddle's Island realized that their small experiment might have meant as much to research methodology as the efficacy of smallpox vaccine meant to public health.

REFERENCES

1. Jenner E. *An Inquiry Into the Causes and Effects of Variolae Vaccinae, a Disease Discovered in Some of the Western Counties of England, Particularly Gloucestershire, and Known by the Name of Cowpox*. London: Sampson Low; 1798.
2. Hopkins DR. *Princes and Peasants: Smallpox in History*. Chicago: The University of Chicago Press; 1983.
3. Winkelstein WJ. Not just a country doctor: Edward Jenner, scientist. *Epidemiologic Reviews* 1992:14; 1–15.

4. Gordon MB, M.D. *Aesculapius Comes to the Colonies: The Story of the Early Days of Medicine in the Thirteen Original Colonies.* New York: Ventnor; 1949.

5. Report of the Board of Health, Boston: Boston Board of Health; December 16, 1802.

6. Diehl HS, Baker AB, Cowen DW. Cold vaccines: an evaluation based on a controlled study. *JAMA* 1938:111; 1168-1173.

7. Blake JB. *Benjamin Waterhouse and the Introduction of Vaccination: A Reappraisal.* Philadelphia: University of Pennsylvania Press; 1957.

8. Woodward S, Feemster R. The relation of smallpox morbidity to vaccination laws. *New Engl Jour Med.* 1933; 208:317–318.

9. Fenner FMD, Arita I, M.D., Henderson DA, M.D., Jezek Z, M.D., Ladnyi ID, M.D. *Smallpox and its Eradication.* Geneva: World Health Organization; 1988.

10. Trent JC. *Benjamin Waterhouse (1754-1846).* Annals of Medical History New York: Henry Schuman; 1946.

CHAPTER 4

Scourge of the Middle West: Autumnal Fever and Daniel Drake

The weather, during the first three weeks of the month of May, was dry and temperate, with now and then a cold day and night. The strawberries were ripe on the 15th, and cherries on the 22nd, day of the month, and in several of the city gardens. A shower of hail fell on the afternoon of the 22nd, which broke the glass windows of many houses. A single stone of this hail was found to weigh two drachms. Several people collected a quantity of it, and preserved it till the next day in their cellars, when they used it for the purpose of cooling their wine.

The weather, after this hail storm, was rainy during the remaining part of the month. The diseases were still inflammatory. Many persons were afflicted with a sore mouth in this month. The weather in June was pleasant and temperate. Several intermittents [fevers] and two very acute pleurisies, occurred in my practice during this month. The intermittents were uncommonly obstinate, and would not yield to the largest doses of the bark. (1, p. 197)

With these words, our friend, Benjamin Rush, began his observations on the diseases that beset Philadelphia in the year following the terrible yellow fever outbreak of 1793. As he had during the epidemic, Rush took pains to observe and catalog weather conditions. His intention was to learn more about disease patterns from clues provided by meteorological factors. These, he was convinced, predisposed to yellow fever and other human illnesses. His correlations, as the text above suggests, were of a general and unsystematic sort. He proclaimed hot, humid weather was unhealthy, noted the summer was the time when fluxes (diarrhea) and fevers were rampant and, as we saw in Chapter 1, praised the cold rains that occurred in mid-October of 1793, as salubrious because they cleansed the air of miasma.

Rush was not alone in his attempt to understand disease by examining the environment. Many in America and abroad were struggling to develop systems that accounted for the phenomena of epidemics. It was natural that they turned to perturbations in the environment for explanations. Weather, climate, geography, and natural surroundings encompass every aspect of human endeavor. Because these elements vary—hot and cold, dry and wet, high and low, windy and still—it was reasonable to assume that relationships might be found between such variations and human health and disease. It was an approach not unlike that of Hippocrates and his extensive catalog of associations between "airs, waters, and places" and the occurrence of illness. Many connections between climate, place, and disease had developed over the centuries since Hippocrates first espoused such principles. Table 4-1 provides a few examples.

One can appreciate the appeal of the approach. Medicine had long struggled for scientific respectability. The discipline was mired in philosophical debates over theories that were centuries old. As the Age of Enlightenment that dominated 18th century Europe thought spread to America, hopes ran high that science, which held such promise for improving human existence, could shake medicine

TABLE 4-1

Historic Associations Between Environmental Conditions and Disease

Environmental Condition	Disease/Health Problem
Marshes/stagnant water	Fever, large spleens
Cold winds	Chest complaints, pleurisy
Rock formations	Kidney and bladder stones
Hot summers	Yellow fever, diarrhea
Decaying waste	Epidemic fevers
Fog and dew	Fevers
Changing weather (hot to cold)	Rheumatism, pneumonia catarrh (colds)

from its doldrums. With the increasing availability of instruments such as the thermometer, barometer, and hygrometer (humidity) came the opportunity to assess the environment in a scientific manner. In the early 19th century, as access to these instruments grew, numbers of medical men began to measure and record aspects of the physical environment in hopes of learning more about the diseases that afflicted their patients.

The effort had some merit. Many observations made during epidemics suggested that there were, indeed, patterns of association. Yellow fever epidemics invariably appeared in summer months and disappeared soon after the autumn frost. Both smallpox and yellow fever first appeared in ports along the eastern seaboard before they spread to the interior of the country. Science might illuminate these relationships and move forward the understanding of disease causation.

Most prominent of the growing group of medical meteorologists was Daniel Drake (see Figure 4-1). Drake was born in New Jersey in 1785, but he was quickly relocated by his westward-wandering family to a frontier outpost just up the Ohio River from Cincinnati. Conditions were primitive in the truest backwoods tradition. The Drakes began their pioneer lives in a one-room, windowless log cabin, with a half-finished wooden chimney and roof that covered one side only. Young Daniel's education was piecemeal at best, provided by itinerant schoolmasters and the minimal library of his modestly literate parents. In addition to the Bible, the almanac, and a chivalric romance, an occasional copy of a local newspaper comprised the literature for his eager mind.

> I recollect getting a number of it [the newspaper] when I was about 11 years old. It was soon after corn planting, and I was sent into the cornfield to keep out the squirrels. I took the paper with me, and leaving the young corn to defend itself as it could, sat down at the root of a large tree near the center of the little field (where of course the squirrels would not disturb me) and, beginning at the head of the first column, on the first page, read it though—advertisements and all. This may seem to you rather laughable, but it was all right (the neglect of corn excepted) for it gave me a peep into the world & and excited my curiosity. (2, pp. 166–167)

Drake labored against the forest with axes, mauls, and plows till the age of 15, when he was sent to apprentice with Dr. William Goforth, a family friend and physician who practiced in Cincinnati.

FIGURE 4-1

Daniel Drake

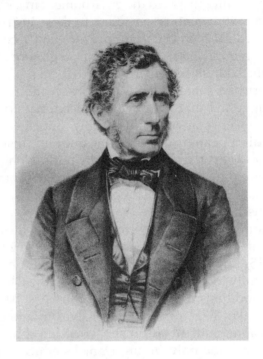

Source: National Library of Medicine.

Following a 5-year apprenticeship, an interval in practice, and a 6-month pilgrimage to Philadelphia to attend lectures by doctors Wistar, Physick, and Woodhouse and the famous Dr. Rush, he settled in the Ohio Valley as teacher and medical practitioner.

Drake earned distinction as a medical educator and public-spirited citizen. In addition to founding the Medical College of Ohio in Cincinnati and the *Western Journal of Medical and Physical Sciences*, he supplied Ohio with its nickname and state tree, the buckeye, in tribute to the many samples of the species he cut down in his youth. He was a man of endless enthusiasms and an avid observer of the physical environment of the Ohio Valley. His first paper, published in 1808, was on "The Epidemic Diseases which Prevail at Mays-Lick in Kentucky," the area in which he lived. It was, like many efforts of the time, composed of two largely independent lists. The first described the characteristics of an outbreak of fever (probably typhoid) which "prevailed in every house in the village."

> The majority were attacked between the 1st and 10th or 15th of October....
> In November and December it (the fever) was attended with more typhus symptoms than in September and October....Pains in the extremities were very common. They were sometimes periodical....Occasional chills were not uncommon.

The second presented unconnected observations of "circumstances which were attendant upon it (the epidemic)":

> The summer and autumn were remarkably dry. Almost every spring was exhausted. The wheat ripened nearly two weeks earlier than usual; and whole fields of corn were destroyed. Almost every different kind of tree defoliated much earlier than usual; and the leaves of some were dried up without assuming those beautiful colours that precede their fall....In proportion to the number of showers which fell, we had very little lightning and thunder....There was, I think, more east-wind than usual....Several different species of insect were uncommonly numerous. (3, pp. 2–4)

Unfortunately, the exact relationship between the outbreak and his environmental observations escaped Drake, who admitted, "I do not pretend to see any connection, after the manner of cause and effect, between these facts and our little epidemic, but, as I cannot assign any cause for it, and as these occurrences were all contemporary, I thought them worth mentioning." Then, confident that the method had potential, he added, "Evils often seem gregarious" (3, p. 4).

Drake developed more extensive projects, cataloging the topography (the soils, rocks, woods, and waters), temperature, and flora around Cincinnati and attempting to relate those to health and disease. His connections grew more specific, but they still offered little that was new. He noted, for example, that "fog and dew appear to precipitate fevers, changing weather from heat to cold (rather than cold to heat) incites rheumatism, tonsillitis, catarrh (colds), and pneumonia, decaying waste is a certain cause of epidemic fevers, and well water containing carbonic acid aids dyspepsia" (3, pp. 29–36).

His culminating and best-remembered work was an ambitious, comprehensive catalog of the diseases that afflicted the middle of America. It was called a *Systematic Treatise, Historical, Etiological, and Practical, on the Principles Diseases of the Interior Valley of North America*, composed of two volumes, of 878 and 985 pages, respectively. Volume 1, published in 1850, was an exhaustive recitation of the topography and climatic characteristics of a vast stretch of America reaching from the Gulf of Mexico to the St. Lawrence River. It also included physiologic and social characteristics of the people who occupied the territory. The second volume, published in 1854, two years after Drake's death, catalogued diseases of the region, their characteristics and presumed causes, as well as treatment. The *Treatise* was a mix of Drake's personal observations and collected scholarship. In preparing the books, he traveled 30,000 miles over 10 years, covering much of the Mississippi Valley, the Great Lakes, and even Lower Canada. He was an exhaustive and eloquent observer of the land and its people:

> The distance between (Bloomington and Peoria) is about forty miles....For the first ten miles, the rolling prairies are interspersed with narrow belts of wood-land, along the head streams of Kickapoo and Sugar Creeks,—waters which belong to the Sangamon Basin. Diluvial or post-tertiary deposits of sand, gravel, and clay, with erratic boulders, bury up the carboniferous rocks. The sparse population is moderately affected with autumnal fever. Passing beyond the waters of Sugar Creek, we come on the dividing lands between it and Mackinaw Creek, a tributary of the Illinois. For many miles this tract presents a high, rolling, argillaceous surface, with scattered oak trees and prairie herbage, to the village of Mackinaw, on the western side of which is the creek of that name. The physician of the village, Doctor Burns, who had formerly resided on White River, in the State of Indiana, told me, that there was autumnal fever "here and there." (4, p. 323)
>
> Our boys begin the use of tobacco, by chewing or smoking, at an early age; many as early as seven years; a large number before puberty; and a great majority of all who ever use it, acquire the habit before they are twenty-one....At whatever period the habit may be formed, it generally continues through life; and the earlier it is established, the more inveterate is its character. The predisposing cause of this custom is the constitutional desire for bodily excitement;...The most efficient exciting cause is fashion, and instinctive imitation of our seniors and companions. (4, p. 674)

The *Treatise* represented a significant advance in Drake's efforts to link environment and disease. Where earlier publications lacked convincing associations between the physical features of the landscape, climate, and disease, Drake now used actual measurements and detailed observations to test specific hypotheses. The disease that Drake attacked with greatest vigor was the one that had by far the greatest social and economic impact on the region. In his travels, he saw its specter in the pale, haunted faces of citizens in town after town. It was known as "the ague" or "autumnal fever."

Autumnal fever was the plague of America's interior. Unlike the outbreaks of yellow fever and smallpox that swept the seaboard cities in terrifying waves, then vanished, to reappear years later, autumnal fever was an omnipresent menace. It was *endemic* rather than epidemic, smoldering continuously along the towns of the Ohio and Mississippi rivers, their tributaries, and on lowland farms from Louisiana to Minnesota. The illness itself was also different. Smallpox and yellow fever produced dramatic episodes of brief duration. After several weeks the outcome would be determined. Such was not the case with autumnal fever, although at first it seemed just like so many other fevers. Patients complain of headache, increasing fatigue, muscle pains, nausea, and fever—as with "the flu" or a multitude of intestinal afflictions. The episode is brief. In several days the temperature returns to normal and recovery appears at hand.

Then something unexpected happens: The disease returns—and recurs not only with much greater force but in repeating episodes. Three stages characterize each recurrence. The first, a *cold stage*, begins with a sudden chill, a feeling of intense cold and uncontrolled shivering. Teeth clatter and the body shakes. Victims try to compensate by bundling on extra clothes or enveloping themselves in blankets. This cold phase isn't long; often it subsides within an hour. A *hot stage* follows, during which the chill is driven out by intense heat. The face grows flushed, the skin dry and burning. A racing pulse and splitting headache are common. The temperature may rise to 106°F or more. The hot stage can last upwards of 6 hours and is, in turn, followed by a *sweating stage*, in which clothes and bedding are drenched by unrelenting perspiration. The body temperature falls rapidly, often to below-normal levels. By now, patients are exhausted and succumb to deep sleep. The total duration of the tripartite attack is relatively short. Symptoms often begin in the afternoon and the entire cycle is completed in 12 hours. Within 24 hours, victims are frequently returned to a reasonably normal condition.

Then it all happens again. Two or three days later the ordeal repeats, with exactly the same sequence: cold stage, hot stage, and

then the drenching sweats. Misery. Recurrences can go on with dia-
bolic regularity for weeks, months, even years—uncanny in their
predictability. Sometimes the illness appears to abate, only to
return months later when the cycle begins again.

Over time such relentless bouts of illness extract a toll, both on
individuals and on whole communities. Hippocrates was actually
describing autumnal fever when he reported on the health of people who lived near stagnant marshes: "[They] have large and firm
spleens while their bellies are hard, warm, and thin. Their shoulders, the parts about the clavicles and their faces are thin too
because their spleens dissolve their flesh" (5, p. 94). Inhabitants of
the Mississippi Valley were similarly depicted centuries later.

> As we drew near Burlington [Iowa] in front of a little hut on the river bank,
> sat a girl and a lad—most pitiable looking objects, uncared for, hollow
> eyed, sallow faced. They had crawled out into the warm sun with chatter-
> ing teeth to see the boat pass. To Mother's inquiries the captain said: "If
> you've never seen that kind of sickness I reckon you must be a Yankee.
> That's the ague. I'm feared you will see plenty of it if you stay long in these
> parts. They call it here the swamp devil and it will take the roses out of the
> cheeks of these plump little ones of yours mighty quick. Cure it? No,
> Madam, No cure for it: have to wear it out. I had it a year when I first went
> on the river." (4, p. xix)

The fever dictated daily existence. Another observer recorded,
"the minister made his appointments to preach so as to accommo-
date his shakes," and "the Justice of the Peace entered the suit on his
docket to avoid the sick day of the party or his own" (6, p. 17). One
distinguished visitor, traveling by riverboat to the confluence of the
Ohio and Mississippi rivers, offered a most unflattering description:

> At the junction of the two rivers, on ground so flat and low and marshy, that
> at certain seasons of the year it is inundated to the house-tops, lies a breed-
> ing-place of fever, ague and death; A dismal swamp, on which the half-built
> houses rot away: cleared here and there for the space of a few yards; and
> teeming, then, with rank, unwholesome vegetation, in whose baleful shade
> the wretched wanderers who are tempted hither, droop, and die, and lay
> their bones. (7, p. 171)

Charles Dickens was only too happy to depart the pale, hollow-
cheeked inmates and the penetrating mosquitoes of Cairo, Illinois
(see Figure 4-2).

FIGURE 4-2

Autumnal Fever Territory

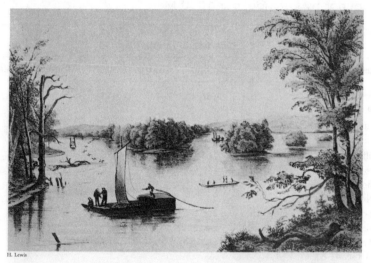

Plate 61. THE MOUTH OF THE MISSOURI RIVER

Source: From a print by Lewis, Library of Congress.

Drake deployed his best science to determine the origins of autumnal fever. Borrowing from army surveys, he produced measurements to identify patterns of disease. Finally, he had data to inform his theories. Tables 4-2 and 4-3 document several attributes of the fever. Worthy of its name, autumnal fever displays a decidedly seasonal pattern. In each of the military posts, cases of fever are lowest in the winter (first quarter of the year) and highest in the summer and early fall (third quarter), as Table 4-2 illustrates. Equally revealing is the distribution of autumnal fever by latitude: The further north one travels from Fort Jackson near the Gulf Coast, the less (for the most part) the occurrence of fever. When one reaches Fort Brady near the shores of Lake Superior, the ague occurs with only a fraction of the frequency of the Mississippi delta. What is it about seasons and latitude that relates to the occurrence of disease? In a second table (see Table 4-3 on page 79), Drake adds temperature measurements. We now can see that temperature influences frequency.

TABLE 4-2

Attacks of Autumnal Fever in Different Quarters of the Year at Military Posts Between the Gulf of Mexico and Lake Superior by Latitude, per 1000 Men

| Posts | Quarters of the Year | | | | |
	First	Second	Third	Fourth	Total of the Year
Fort Jackson, N. Lat. 29 29'	86	157	944	413	1600
Baton Rouge, N. Lat. 30 36'	111	186	320	207	824
Jefferson Barracks, N. Lat. 38 28'	48	80	228	119	475
Fort Leavenworth, N. Lat. 39 20'	101	154	221	153	629
Fort Armstrong, N. Lat. 41 28'	15	100	145	47	307
Fort Dearborn, N. Lat. 41 51'	10	67	106	68	251
Fort Crawford, N. Lat. 43 3'	13	42	172	72	301
Fort Howard, N. Lat. 44 40'	4	17	50	13	84
Fort Snelling, N. Lat. 44 53'	2	12	34	14	62
Fort Brady, N. Lat. 46 39'	1	16	22	5	44

Source: Based on Drake (4), pp. 706–707. (Table shortened for illustrative purposes.)

Cases decline as one moves northward—from an average annual temperature of 68 degrees in Baton Rouge, Louisiana, to 57 at the Jefferson Barracks near St. Louis, to the chilly 45 and readings at Fort Snelling near Minneapolis.

To the measurements of season, latitude, and temperature, Drake adds his observations on two topographical features: water and soil. Surface water is particularly suspect. He documents that in places where pools of standing water are abundant, autumnal fever is rife; where the landscape is dry, the disease is virtually unrecognized.

TABLE 4-3

Attacks of Autumnal Fever by Latitude and Average Annual Temperature at Military Posts Along the Mississippi River Between the Gulf of Mexico and Lake Superior, per 1000 Men

Posts	Fever Cases	Average Annual Temperature, in °F
Baton Rouge, N. Lat. 30 36'	824	68
Jefferson Barracks, N. Lat. 38 28'	475	57
Fort Armstrong, N. Lat. 41 28'	307	51
Fort Crawford, N. Lat. 43 3'	301	47
Fort Snelling, N. Lat. 44 53'	62	45

Source: Based on Drake (4), p. 713. (Table shortened for illustrative purposes.)

As we ascend the Mississippi, to the mouth of the Missouri, we find its annual floods leaving small ponds, swamps, and lagoons; which in the aggregate, are of great extent, and but partially drained or dried up, before the next inundation. Now, as we have seen, the whole of this region is infested with autumnal fever, beyond any other portion of the valley.

In the states of Illinois, Indiana and Ohio, the rivers generally flow through wide valleys, any of which, are liable to be overflowed. Small lakes, ponds and swamps, are also frequent...and it is precisely these localities, which are most infested. To the east of all the states mentioned, as we climb the mountains, the surface water is no longer found in basins; and the streams, generally, have a rapid current, down narrow and rocky channels; and here, autumnal fever nearly disappears...Everywhere, west of the states of Arkansas, Missouri, and Iowa, surface water is scarce.... Thus, as we advance into that desert, we come at the same time to the limits of surface water, and of autumnal fever." (4, p. 711)

The organic content of soil is a third factor that Drake believes breeds the ague.

Now, it is a safe generalization to affirm that, all other circumstances being equal, autumnal fever prevails most where the amount of organic matter is greatest, and least where it is least.... Decaying organic matter is *one* of the conditions necessary to the production of autumnal fever. (4, p. 709)

These three characteristics—warm temperature, standing water, and organic matter in the soil—are all associated with autumnal fever. But how exactly do the elements create disease? Are they themselves sufficient to cause illness? Or do they promote or enable other agents, such as miasmas or noxious gasses or, as had been suggested by occasional mavericks dating back as far as Cotton Mather, living, microscopic particles or animalcules?

Drake recognizes there are three hypotheses competing for medical and popular support. He brings his observations to bear on each possibility, one at a time. The first, the meteoric hypothesis, is the view that heat and humidity are sufficient to produce autumnal fever. Drake has data that support this notion—the links between warm, moist environments and the occurrence of fever. But he also has observations that challenge the hypothesis and render it an insufficient explanation for autumnal fever:

> It is well known, that autumnal fever seldom appears on board of vessels which cruise in the Gulf of Mexico, although the air, at the temperature of eighty, is nearly saturated with vapour.
>
> The sandy banks of Pensacola Bay, from its entrance, up to the town of Pensacola, suffer but little; while, at the head of the bay, where extensive alluvial deposits have been made, the Fever has been so constant and fatal as to prevent permanent settlements. Yet the temperature and moisture of both localities are the same, for they are but ten miles apart.
>
> Lastly, in some of our manufacturing establishments, the in-door artisans and operatives, labor in a heated atmosphere supersaturated with vapor, but remain free from autumnal fever. (4, pp. 717–718)

The second theory he calls the "malarial hypothesis." This holds that the noxious gasses, or *mal-arias* (bad air), that arise from decaying organic matter in the earth are responsible. It is, of course, little more than of Benjamin Rush's miasmas made scientific by the terminology of medical meteorology. Drake's catalog of rock formations and subsoils across the geographic expanse where autumnal fever prevails supports the observation that illness is more frequent in regions where the soil is rich in organic matter. Gasses arising from this material would seem a plausible explanation for disease. But Drake again counters his own findings by noting inconsistencies: "It is well known to us all, that there are sickly and healthy seasons at the same place, and sometimes over large portions of our Valley, while the amount of organic matter remains unchanged" (4, p. 722).

This leaves one more theory: the *animalcular hypothesis*. "The microscope has revealed the existence of a countless variety of organic forms," Drake reports, "which surround and penetrate the bodies of larger animals and plants, whether living or dead, and decaying, inhabit all waters, salt and fresh, and swarm in the atmosphere" (4, p. 723). These, he believes, can creep upon us as invisibly as noxious gases and impart disease without being seen. As water, high temperature, and abundant vegetation are likely to favor the development of living organisms, their higher prevalence in warm and humid climates would be no surprise. Other facts support this hypothesis:

> We know that water is essential to the support of those animal and veg-etable forms which are matters of observation by the unassisted eye; and may conclude, therefore, that it is equally necessary for the tribes which are invisible.
>
> A high temperature is favorable to the development of animal and veg-etable life. In the southern parts of the Valley, animal forms, especially of the lower order, are greatly multiplied, and vegetation is luxuriant. If this be true of the visible, why may we not conclude that it is equally true of the invisible? Now, it is precisely in those regions, that the Fever, other circum-stances being equal, displays its greatest prevalence and malignity. (4, pp. 724–725)

Finally, he concludes: "From what has been said, it appears obviously, I think, that the etiological history of autumnal fever, can be more successfully explained by the...animalcular hypothe-sis, than the malarial" (4, p. 727).

Drake creates an argument for disease causation of far greater scientific plausibility than had been seen before in America. The process is impressive. He first collects a set of relevant facts. He then makes explicit comparisons to create correlations, associations between the environmental factors and disease: Autumnal fever occurs in a seasonal pattern. Cases are far more frequent in summer and early autumn compared with the colder months of the year. Disease is also far more common in the south compared with the north. The fever is clearly linked with environmental warmth; dis-ease rates decrease when the average temperature drops and are more prevalent where there is standing water and organic soil.

He establishes that temperature, surface water, and soil are critical factors, then challenges existing theories. Sifting the assem-bled facts, he probes to see where confirmation sits and inconsis-tency lies. Do current theories stand up to the spectrum of evidence?

Is autumnal fever brought on by the actions of heat and humidity alone: the meteoric hypothesis? Or do the heat and humidity simply act on organic matter in the soil to create noxious gases, the miasmas Rush believed emanated from decaying organic matter, the *mal-arias* the Greeks and Romans saw as seeping from the stinking swamps? Or do warm, moist environments and organic soils interact to spawn invisible, microscopic organisms?

Drake sides with the microorganisms. They fit with the climate data and hold up better to the challenge of his additional observations.* The methods are a great advance. Where most American doctors of the time were still relying on untested theories of disease, Drake had gathered data and used them to confront prevailing ideology. He had uncovered the strength of an approach that lies in utilizing both confirming and refuting evidence. It is a process that is still in use today. One currently used criterion for supporting the causal nature of an association is the finding that data from a variety of different settings from different researchers using different methods all point to the same conclusion. Others rely on refutation. A 20th-century philosopher of science named Karl Popper, for one, argues that scientific hypotheses can only be refuted, and never proven (8). Regardless of the amount of data that support the theory that malaria occurs only below the latitude of 50 degrees, one can never be certain that such a case will not occur. Should it happen, however, the refutation of the theory would be compelling.

Drake had hoped his studies would reveal the cause of autumnal fever. But as he sorted the data and confronted the varying hypotheses, he found that the puzzle was still incomplete.

His correlations between characteristics of the environment and autumnal fever appeared to be on target, but he had not yet pinpointed the direct cause for the disease. More pieces were needed. How exactly did autumnal fever come about? What was it about heat and humidity that produced disease? If there were animalcules involved, how did they gain access to the body? How was the cyclic nature of fevers explained? Some details were missing. While there was clearly a correlation between climate and the ague, there was more to the story.

---

* He was not the first to propose this theory. Others had espoused the idea many years earlier, including Cotton Mather.

From the vantage point of the 21st century, the story is much clearer, if no less complex. Drake was correct—at least in part. Autumnal fever was caused by a microorganism, a tiny living particle that proliferated in the human body and brought on the recurrent fevers, the swollen spleens, and the chronic wasting so characteristic of the condition. It was almost 30 years after Drake's treatise first appeared when the puzzle came together. In 1880, a French military doctor named Alphonse Charles Laveran, working in Algeria, saw through his microscope peculiar, pigmented bodies in the blood of fever sufferers. These turned out to be the very animalcules that Drake thought might be there. They were the direct, or, in Drake's terminology, "efficient" cause of the disease: simple, single cells that were given the name *Plasmodium*. Plasmodia initiate a chain of events that culminates in autumnal fever when they enter the human blood stream, invade red blood cells, feed on the cell's oxygen carrying protein known as hemoglobin, and multiply. From 10 to 20 of these miniscule parasites can grow within a single red cell before their burden exceeds the capacity of the red cell and the cell explodes. When this occurs among many cells, millions of plasmodia flood the bloodstream. There they seek out new red cell homes in which to feed and multiply, only to burst forth again when their growth exceeds the cells' ability to shelter them.

Each time a red cell ruptures, it releases not only new parasites but a variety of cellular enzymes and proteins. It is these substances to which the body responds with fever. The process of cell invasion, growth, and rupture takes 2 to 3 days. The cycle then repeats again and again. Over several weeks, the cycles of millions of rupturing cells occur synchronously, and the characteristic 2- to 3-day pattern of chills, fever, and sweating is born. But these debilitating episodes are only part of the problem. The destruction of red blood cells is another. As the disease progresses and red cells are lost, patients grow anemic. Tissues of the body become starved of their needed oxygen and energy is sapped. Patients grow listless and defeated. Throughout all this, the immune system struggles to contain the infection. Immune cells engulf and destroy invading parasites. Many of these defensive cells reside in the spleen and, as the battle proceeds, the spleen enlarges to meet the challenge— the explanation for the swollen abdomens so prevalent in regions where the ague prevails. In previously healthy individuals, the parasites may be defeated in a matter of weeks. Among people who are poorly nourished or have immunity that is depleted from other conditions, the disease may go on for months, adding burden to an already weakened system. Recovery is not always the outcome. The disease can be fatal and is especially hazardous for pregnant women and infants.

Autumnal fever is not contagious. The disease is not transmitted directly from person to person as, so obviously, is smallpox. Nor is it spread by heat-induced disorders of the atmosphere or by noxious miasmas rising from decaying refuse. It was not until the closing years of the 19th century that an Englishman named Ronald Ross, laboring in the heat of India, using painstaking techniques of microscopic dissection, found the final piece. He discovered the *Plasmodium* parasite in the salivary gland of an insect. Autumnal fever—the terrible ague that not only had ravaged the Mississippi Valley but had, for centuries, created mayhem around the planet—depended upon a common household pest for its proliferation. Mosquitoes spread it.

The particular culprit is a breed of mosquito known as *Anopheles* (see Figure 4-3). *Anopheles* is only one of a number of mosquito

FIGURE 4-3

Anopheles Mosquito

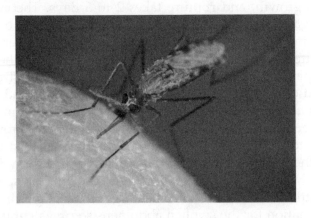

Source: James Gathany, courtesy Centers for Disease Control and Prevention.

types (genera). Among the group are several hundred species. Only a small proportion of these carries Plasmodia and feeds on humans. Those that do, become infected when they extract a "blood meal" from a person who already has parasites circulating in his or her blood. Parasites within infected red cells are liberated inside the mosquito's stomach. The parasite completes a reproductive cycle within the mosquito, eventually producing thousands of fibrous *sporozoites*, which migrate to the mosquito's salivary glands (where Ross discovered them). From there they are injected into the unsuspecting person the mosquito chooses for its next meal. Only the female *Anopheles* sucks human blood. Males are vegetarians, content to feed on fruits and flowers. The female feeds voraciously, often ingesting more than twice her own weight in blood at a single meal. But her gluttony is a selfless act. The blood meal is taken only in the interest of her progeny. She, like the male, could exist without animal blood. Her need for protein-rich hemoglobin is to produce her brood. These future pests (as many as 500) are deposited as eggs on the surfaces of ponds, puddles, or almost any collection of undisturbed water. The variety of these aqueous nurseries is almost limitless, and differing types of mosquitoes have particular preferences. Some varieties prefer to breed in swamps and ponds of the woodlands and countryside. Others are urban dwellers and breed in the midst of human habitation—in rain barrels, tin cans, flower vases, and abandoned auto tires. The eggs hatch into tiny larvae, which rest just beneath the surface of the water, breathing through tiny tubes that barely break the surface. After a typical interval of 10 days or so and several moltings, the adult mosquito is ready to leave the water, ready to mate, and ready to find a victim to bite.

It is a complicated piece of science with an ironic twist. While the remarkable discoveries of the late 19th century proved the final knell for the miasma theory, the newly described disease was not to be shed of its oldest association. It was called *malaria.*

The associations Drake worked so hard to uncover did hold up in the light of new knowledge. The disease prospered in warm, moist climates, where milder seasons meant longer periods for mosquitoes to breed and feed before the cold weather shut down activity. His correlations with locations where standing water was plentiful were also confirmed. The marshes, ponds, and pools were necessary breeding sites for the *Anopheles* mosquito.* Although Drake failed to pinpoint a single, "efficient" cause for autumnal fever, it is difficult to fault him. The idea of finding a unitary, direct cause for every disease is appealing. It boasts economy and simplicity—oversimplicity. The logical appeal does not fit with the realities.

The more we learn about diseases, the more complex the concept of causation becomes. Often there are multiple factors that operate at different levels of proximity to the outcome. Malaria is an excellent example. Many elements play a role in the affliction. Each contributes in some fashion to producing the disease in humans. But some are clearly more directly related than others. Several of the elements are absolutely necessary—the parasite, *Plasmodium*, for example. Without *Plasmodium* in the bloodstream, there would be no illness. At the same time, without *Anopheles* mosquitoes, there would be no *Plasmodium* in the bloodstream. And without standing water for breeding and temperatures warm enough to support procreation, there would be no *Anopheles* mosquitoes. Without human reservoirs of parasites, there would be no source for a large supply of the *Plasmodium*. And so it goes. The interlocking components are extensive.

But other associations—other characteristics of the environment—though less obviously causal, are also important. Several connect the occurrence of fever with environmental changes that accompanied America's westward expansion. It was noted, for example, that prior to the clearing and cultivating of new land, when only a few settlers occupied the uncut forest, good health prevailed. There was little fever among the inhabitants. It was only when clearing began, the trees were felled, roads and homesteads carved out, the trappings of development begun that life became unhealthy; the ague appeared. Once the land passed through this phase and into stable cultivation, salubrity returned. Said Drake: "The first breaking up of the soil appears, from a variety of observation, scattered through our topographical descriptions, to be frequently followed

---

* In fact, Drake had nearly stumbled upon the critical puzzle piece when he observed in the *Treatise* that "autumnal fever prevails very unequally in different years.... In the same locality, it may, in one autumn be malignant and epidemic, and in another mild and sporadic...[just as] it has often happened that mosquitoes have been absent from the banks of the middle portion of the Ohio river for a year, and in the next appear in immense numbers" (4, p. 726).

by autumnal fever; and, on the other hand, long-continued cultivation is accompanied by diminution of that disease"(4, p. 710).

The pattern was so commonly observed that people accepted the predicted fluctuations in health as part of the cost of settlement. They even named the strange phenomenon. It was known as *seasoning the land*.

Once the complex picture of malaria was completed, "seasoning" could be explained. The sequential changes to the landscape had a direct impact on the Anopheles mosquito. Before the land was cleared, mosquitoes viewed the deeply shaded woodlands as inhospitable for breeding. Anopheles prefers to lay its eggs in water where they receive sunlight. Once the trees are felled, existing ponds and pools become exposed. In addition, as the land is civilized, new ponds are built, and water collects in depressions in the landscape created by clearing rocks and stumps. The activity creates new habitat, not just for humans, but for their insect adversaries. After some years, when stable cultivation comes, mosquito-breeding habitat diminishes. Swampy land is drained to provide additional acreage for crops. Livestock is brought in—this to the delight of the mosquitoes, which, it turns out, prefer pigs and cattle to humans as a source of blood meals.

Changing characteristics of the host also contribute. During active periods of human migration, malaria spreads. Individuals with chronic plasmodial infections carry their parasites with them when they move to new communities. Susceptible newcomers are fresh hosts. The greater the human movement from place to place, the more malaria prospers. As communities stabilize, and the population weathers the disease and grows immune, the frequency of disease declines. As communities become settled, better housing is built and nutrition improves. Tighter houses mean less access for mosquitoes; a better-nourished populace is better equipped to develop immunity to the disease.

The miasmatists, like Rush and those who followed him, intimated an understanding of the complexities of causal relationships. They theorized that both the disordered atmosphere and predisposing human factors were required before epidemic disease, such as yellow fever, could occur. Such had to be the case. To reconcile the observations that not everyone who was exposed to the same noxious environment, who breathed the same air, became ill, required mitigating factors. Other elements had to work in concert with the miasmas to create illness. Predisposing human failings, such as poverty, lack of cleanliness, inadequate moral fiber, and the like were logical candidates. Since many of the diseases of the 19th century, including fevers, occurred most often in poor, crowded neighborhoods, where not only a lack of cleanliness, but "immorality" were all too evident, there was support for the notion.

Though many "secondary" elements seem less-directly related in the causal picture of malaria, they demonstrate a critical property of a causal relationship. The elimination of any one may interrupt the transmission of disease. This test turns out to be a critical determinant in our ideas about causation. If an element or factor is removed from the pattern, does the disease cease to exist? In the case of malaria, elimination of the parasite, the mosquito, the mosquito's breeding habitat, or infected hosts upon whom mosquitoes feed will break the transmission of disease. Understanding the intricate pattern of malaria transmission, and specifically identifying characteristics that are critical in the causal path, do more than simply satisfy our etiologic curiosity. They suggest opportunities for intervention. Thoughts about preventing *mal-aria* existed long before Laveran and Ross announced their discoveries. Hippocrates' Greeks appreciated that avoiding marshy areas and eschewing romantic walks in the evening air lessened one's chances of contracting fever (the areas and the time of day when feeding mosquitoes were most prevalent).

With understanding of the interrelationships between the human host, the insect vector, the parasite, and the environment come opportunities to break the cycle. Appreciating the habits of the mosquito and eliminating or reducing aqueous breeding sites is one series of options. Reducing contact with human hosts by protective screening is another. More recent, and more controversial, approaches have relied on the use of chemicals, both as insecticides to kill mosquitoes and as repellents to prevent their interaction with the human hosts.

Malaria was at its worst in the Mississippi Valley during the middle of the 19th century. Death rates from the disease peaked about 1850, then, declined dramatically over 50 years, so that by the early decades of the 20th century, cases were reported on a sporadic basis only in Iowa, Minnesota, Wisconsin, and Illinois. This was not the situation in the southern United States. Malaria continued to beset the south. It was not until after the conclusion of the Second World War, after troops had been brought home and resettled, that the entire country was considered free of the disease.

The decline of autumnal fever occurred well in advance of any systematic efforts to eradicate it. Long before 20th-century initiatives that aggressively attacked the *Anopheles* by draining marshes, pouring suffocating oil on ponds, and lavishing DDT, rates of malaria were falling. While reasons for the decline are not certain, it appears they to relate to changes in the environment. Malaria was a part of a changing ecology. Conditions no longer favored the *Anopheles* or her *Plasmodia* parasites. The stabilization of population migration into cities and towns, mature farming practices that drained land for cultivation and brought livestock close to human habitation to provide tasty alternatives for the mosquitoes, and a rising prosperity that brought improved housing and better nourishment all contributed to the eradication of malaria from the United States.

The success of the U.S. experience with malaria is not reflected in the rest of the world. There are still large expanses of South America, sub-Saharan Africa, and Southeast Asia that remain affected—about 100 countries in all. Several billion people are at constant risk from the disease. It is estimated that between 300 and 500 million clinical cases occur each year, primarily in Africa, and claim between 1 and 2 million lives. Many of the deaths are in children below the age of 5. Nor is the pattern of occurrence static. Malaria has reemerged in areas where once it had been eradicated and has increased in epidemic proportions where it had existed in a stable, endemic form. Not surprisingly, areas with political unrest or armed conflict where large numbers of refugees have moved from place to place have spawned outbreaks of the disease. Mining, logging, and other development in South America and Southeast Asia, where forests are cut and large groups of nonimmune workers migrate in, has also, like the westward expansion in early America, led to increases in malaria.

The passion for measuring meteoric conditions and recording geography in an effort to understand disease waned as the 1900s wore on—replaced by the discovery of the very germs that Drake had anticipated. The contributions of Laveran and Ross were, of course, part of this "brave new world."

Still, Drake's efforts should not be discounted. The interplay he documented between host and environment in the creation of illness has proven an enduring insight. It is now standard wisdom that detailing the relationships between hosts, the agents that afflict them, and the environment is essential to understanding the production and remedy of disease. Drake's attempt to provide a numeric basis on which to demonstrate these relationships was a great advance over the generalized theories of the miasmatists. His carefully recorded observations, together with his technique of using facts both to defend and attack, support and refute prevailing theories foreshadowed current approaches to testing causal theories.

His *Treatise* remains impressive, not simply in ambition but as prelude to the bacteriologic revolution and to more contemporary methods of scientific inquiry. Drake's search for information was remarkable, taking him from the Great Lakes to the Gulf of Mexico. Still, much of his text was of necessity based on the work of others. No single individual could have hoped to capture the vast territory he set out to catalogue. And, despite his commitment to numbers, the *Treatise* was still light on quantitative measures. The best data he provides are those actually compiled by a young Army officer named Samuel Forry some years earlier. Notably absent is an enumeration of cases of disease or deaths from particular afflictions.

But the lack of such specifics was a deficiency that extended well beyond Drake. It was a national issue. No numeric approaches to solving health problems, including medical meteorology, could succeed without a system of vital statistics that captured consistent information on important health events. It was not until beyond the midpoint of the 19th century, as we shall see in the next chapter, that such need received attention. By that time, Daniel Drake's contribution was complete.

REFERENCES

1. Rush B. *Medical Inquiries and Observations.* Vol. 3, 4th ed. Philadelphia: Griggs & Dickinsons; 1815.

2. Drake D. *Pioneer Life in Kentucky 1785–1800*. New York: Henry Schuman, Inc.; 1948.
3. Shapiro HD, Miller ZL. *Physician to the West: Selected Writings of Daniel Drake on Science & Society*. Lexington: University of Kentucky; 1970.
4. Drake D, Levine ND. *Malaria in the Interior Valley of North America*. Urbana: University of Illinois Press; 1964.
5. Chadwick J, Mann WN. *The Medical Work of Hippocrates*. Oxford: Blackwell Scientific; 1950.
6. Ackerknecht EH. *Malaria in the Upper Mississippi Valley 1760–1900*. Baltimore: The John Hopkins Press; 1945.
7. Dickens C. *American Notes and Pictures from Italy*. London: Oxford University Press; 1846.
8. Buck C. Popper's philosophy for epidemiologists. *Int J Epid*. 1975: 4; 159–168.

CHAPTER 5

Improving the Numbers: Lemuel Shattuck's Report

Americans living in the first half of the 19th century were an optimistic lot. Their new country had survived the internal political struggles that followed the Revolution, successfully fended off the British in the War of 1812, and were in possession of vast new territories to the west. Opportunity was everywhere. People were convinced that theirs was the most salubrious of places. When they compared existence in the New World with that in the overcrowded, polluted capitals of Europe, they rejoiced in the promise of fuller, longer, more productive lives. Indeed, such facts as were available supported this belief. Life expectancy in America had increased steadily, and death rates in both countryside and towns of the new republic appeared considerably lower than in Europe. In London, 1 of every 40 inhabitants died each year, as did 1 in every 32 Parisians; in Vienna the figure was 1 in 22. In Concord, Massachusetts, however, the mortality was only 1 in 66 each year (1, p. 226).

The citizens of Massachusetts seemed particularly blessed. They had largely avoided the yellow fever epidemics that had swept east coast communities to their south and, with smallpox vaccination in general use, had escaped outbreaks of that disease for some years. Convinced that they were the beneficiaries of industrious and upright living, they saw the prospects for continuing good health as exceptionally bright.

But as the 19th century neared its midpoint, a disturbing cloud appeared. It seemed that health was no longer improving. Rather, there was evidence of decline. Alarming figures revealed that between the first and fourth decades of the century, average life expectancy in the towns of Boston, Philadelphia, and New York had fallen. In Boston, the average length of life had dropped by almost 7 years. For a particularly vulnerable portion of the population, children less than 5 years of age, the percentage dying each year had risen from 6% in 1830 to 9% in 1845 (2, p. 104).

This was unexpected news. Its purveyor was an unlikely, unassuming, punctilious Bostonian by the name of Lemuel Shattuck (see Figure 5-1). Unlike our previous heroes—Rush, Boylston, Waterhouse, and Drake—Shattuck was not a physician, but a bookseller. He was an amateur in the health field, without training in science or philosophy, and with little formal education. He began life in Massachusetts in 1793, the year of the great yellow fever epidemic in Philadelphia. His early career was as a schoolteacher. He peregrinated through his 20s from Ipswich, New Hampshire, to Troy, New York, to Detroit,

FIGURE 5-1

Lemuel Shattuck

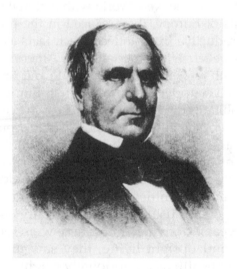

Source: National Library of Medicine.

where he established Michigan's first Sabbath school. Returning to Massachusetts at about the age of 30, he located in Concord. There he resided for 10 years, distinguishing himself as a genealogist and town historian. From Concord he moved to Cambridge and then to Boston, and set up as a bookseller, publisher, genealogist, and public-spirited citizen. He served on the town council, and on two different occasions he was elected to the state legislature. He was described as "a good specimen of a self-made man," a man of deeply moral and religious upbringing. It was, however, also said that "his manner and conversation were very precise and pompous" (3).

Although officially a businessman, Shattuck developed a passion for vital statistics. While writing his history of Concord, he became fascinated by the data he uncovered and by the potential he saw in numbers to illuminate human experience:

> Few subjects are more interesting than accurate bills of mortality. They are the most authentic evidence of the influence of climate and local circumstances on health and human life; and teach a lesson, admonishing us of the destiny that awaits all mankind, and warning us "to live prepared to die." (1, p. 223)

At the same time, Shattuck became acutely aware of the limitations of the data that were available at the time. He found great gaps in the statistics that described the very basics of human existence: birth, marriage, and death. Throughout most of the history of the country, such data were collected haphazardly, if at all. Only when epidemics such as smallpox or yellow fever loomed did interest kindle in collecting numbers to track the health of a community. Once threats to public health abated, the motivation to keep careful records subsided as well. In 1810, the Board of Health of Boston was mandated by the legislature to supervise burials and require a recording of the name, age, sex, and cause of death for each deceased person. Even then results continued to be sporadic, as regulations were not enforced.

Convinced of the value of vital statistics, Shattuck dedicated himself to their improvement. In 1839, he became a founding member of the American Statistical Association. The new association, made up of Shattuck and four others, was patterned after similar, newly emerging organizations in Europe. The prevailing notion of statistics then was not of complex mathematical formulas for testing hypotheses but of practical cataloguing of human events that would serve as the basis for social improvement. Originally, statistics was thought of as "political arithmetic," a gathering and sorting of facts to illuminate the workings (or failings) of the state. The activity appealed to Americans, many of whom had few skills beyond those of simple arithmetic, but who had a zest for describing every aspect of their new country—from its flora and fauna to its weather and its words.

In 1841 Shattuck produced a report called *Vital Statistics of Boston* in which he elaborated in far greater detail than had been done previously mortality data covering a period of 40 years (2). Unlike the disease-specific focus of Drake's descriptions of autumnal fever, Shattuck sought a broader assessment of health. He compiled data on overall patterns of mortality over sequential years, convinced that charting *trends* would produce insights on the origins and, ultimately, the means of preventing disease. His report was innovative. In it Shattuck produces meticulous tables showing the numbers of deaths according to year and by age. The data on mortality displayed in Table 5-1 caused him to despair.

In the table, Shattuck presents the number of deaths that have occurred in 3 intervals of time during the almost 30 years between 1811 and 1839. He also calculates the proportion of all deaths that are contributed by each age category. It is evident that deaths have increased. Most troubling to Shattuck, however, is the growing proportion of deaths occurring in the youngest age group, those under 5 years of age. During the first time interval, from 1811 to 1820, 33.6% of all deaths were among these young children. That proportion is shocking in itself. But over the succeeding intervals, the proportion increases. By 1830–1839 it has grown to 43.1%. Shattuck laments: "It is a melancholy fact, and one which should arrest the attention of all, that 43 per cent or nearly half of all the deaths which have taken place in Boston during the last nine years, are of persons under 5 years of age; and the proportional mortality of this age has been increasing" (2, p. xxiv).

He admonishes his readers that

the causes of this increasing and alarming mortality should be investigated, and, if possible, removed. We have endeavoured to ascertain some of these causes....More luxury and effeminacy in both sexes prevail now than formerly; and this may have had some influence in producing

TABLE 5-1

Deaths and Percent of Deaths by Age in Boston in Three Different Periods of Time

Age	1811–1820		1821–1830		1831–1839	
	Number Dying	Percent of Deaths	Number Dying	Percent of Deaths	Number Dying	Percent of Deaths
Under 5	2698	33.6	3975	37.0	6240	43.1
5 to 10	284	3.6	406	3.8	619	4.3
10 to 20	430	5.4	533	5.0	735	5.1
20 to 30	1133	14.1	1404	13.1	1843	12.7
30 to 40	980	12.2	1392	13.0	1651	11.4
40 to 50	871	10.9	1089	10.2	1156	8.0
50 to 60	560	7.0	720	6.7	821	5.7
60 to 70	456	5.7	520	4.8	646	4.5
70 to 80	386	4.8	429	4.0	496	3.4
80 to 90	193	2.4	229	2.8	225	1.6
90 to 100	29	0.4	37	0.3	51	0.4
Total	8020	100	10731	100	14483	100
Deaths per 100 population	—	2.09	—	2.05	—	2.14

Source: Based on Shattuck (2, p. xxi).

constitutional debility, and the consequent feeble health of children. The nursing and feeding of children with improper food is another cause. The influence of bad air in confined, badly located, and filthy houses is another and perhaps the greatest." (2, p. xxv)

It is an analysis of mixed parts—part scientific and part moral. It typifies Shattuck's approach. Pledged an objective observer, he deplored anything less than the rigorous where matters of gathering evidence were concerned:

We have no sympathy with the opinions of some modern reformers, who seem to be governed by theories founded on uncertain and partial data, or vague conjecture. We are a statist—a dealer in facts. We wish to ascertain the laws of human life, developed by the natural constitution of our bodies, as they actually exist under the influences that surround them, and to learn how far they may be modified and improved. This can only be done by an accurate knowledge of the facts that are daily occurring among us. (4, pp. 21–22)

Interpretation of the data was another matter, however. Like many of his time, Shattuck held strong beliefs that optimal health and moral order were inexorably tied. As a product of the Second Great Awakening, a religious revival that swept through rural New England when he was young, his values were always in evidence:

> The universal thirst for wealth in America, the reckless speculations of some, the hap-hazard mode of living and the disregard to health of others, the luxury and extravagance of certain classes and other practices of modern society—tend to check the progress of the population, increase disease, and weaken the race. (4, p. 22)

The assessment of childhood mortality reflects his conflicting views. Though he acknowledges that environmental and social factors contribute to increased mortality (children's improper feeding and "the influence of bad air in confined, badly located, and filthy houses"), he cannot resist chastising that "more luxury and effeminacy in both sexes prevail now than formerly."

Shattuck was keen not only on charting mortality trends but in identifying the particular diseases responsible. This interest reflected both a growing national acceptance of the notion of disease specificity and his own confidence in the value of identifying patterns of occurrence of particular maladies. But here Shattuck encountered a serious problem. Medical terminology was in disarray. The *classification* of causes of death was completely lacking in consistent usage. Frustrated with attempts to identify the causes of death in his research, he observed:

> The records in this respect are not full and probably they are not always correct in regard to the cause of death....The nomenclature has been several times altered and the disease is often returned one year under a name differing from that of the same disease contained in the return of another year. Even in the same year, one and the same disease often appears under two synonymous names, sometimes under the popular, and sometimes under the scientific name, or under both popular names. (2, p. xxx)

It should come as little surprise that there was inconsistency in nomenclature, given the lack of agreement among the medical profession about the very nature of disease as well as the variable education and training of those who practiced the art. Those who actually recorded the causes of death added more variability to the problem. Since doctors were not required to report deaths (and were often reluctant to admit to adverse outcomes for fear of adverse effects on their practices and incomes), it was often the church sexton or the town clerk who transcribed the cause of death. And the information was usually obtained from grieving family members.

Even when diseases were reported *reliably*-that is, in a consistent manner from one occasion to the next-the *validity*, the true relationship to mortality, was often doubtful. Many attributions would elevate the eyebrows of modern nosologists, (for example, "teething, worms, lethargy, and rash"). Other assigned causes were absurdly vague (for example, "old age, sudden death, mortification, and debility"). Large numbers of childhood deaths were set down to "infantile disease." Other causes were simply signs or symptoms that may accompany a variety of diseases (for example, "jaundice, colic, dyspepsia, spasms").

Shattuck had identified a critical problem, one that plagues us to the present time. One cannot determine trends in the health of any population without accurate information on the diseases involved. One of his principal contributions was the effort to improve classification. Utilizing his position with the American Statistical Association, he enlisted the aid of the newly formed Massachusetts Medical Society. Together they lobbied the Massachusetts General Court (the legislature) to enact laws that would both improve the recording of *vital events*, such as births, deaths, and marriages, and standardize the system of mortality classification.

In this endeavor, he found inspiration in events occurring across the Atlantic in England where there was similar interest in registration of vital events and accurate classification of causes of death. Shattuck had communicated with William Farr, a leader in promoting the passage of a comprehensive, English civil registration law in 1837. Farr had produced a new, advanced system for classifying diseases that he shared with Shattuck. In 1847, Shattuck became a member of the first committee on medical nomenclature created by the newly formed American Medical Association (AMA). At his suggestion, Farr's *nosology*, his system for classifying disease, was adopted by the AMA's national convention. The association summarized the case eloquently:

> No subject which can claim public attention should excite greater interest than that of obtaining a knowledge of the diseases and causes of death in operation among us. It is of great consequence to all of us to know when, where, in what form, and under what circumstances, sickness and mortality take place; and whether they are uniform, or dissimilar in different places, or in the same place in different seasons, and under different circumstances. Wherever this knowledge is possessed, remedies for the amelioration or extinction of existing evils can be applied more intelligently, and with better hope of success. (4, p. 201, appendix IV)

But all this was only a prelude to Shattuck's "master work." Together with colleagues from the Statistical Association and the Medical Society, Shattuck convinced the legislature that a "sanitary survey" of Massachusetts was required:

> By a Sanitary Survey of the State is meant, an examination or survey of the different parts of the Commonwealth,—its counties, its towns, and its localities,—to ascertain the causes which favorably or unfavorably affect the health of its inhabitants. *The word sanitary means relating to health.* When we speak of the sanitary condition of a town, we include a description of those circumstances which relate to, or have an effect upon, the health of its inhabitants. (5, p. 9)

The legislature charged a commission of three members, with Shattuck as its head, to conduct the study. The *Report of the Sanitary Commission of Massachusetts* was published in 1850 and became known as simply "The Shattuck Report" for its principle author. It is a landmark in the history of American public health. The vision that drove the report was extraordinary:

> WE BELIEVE *that the conditions of perfect health, either public or personal, are seldom or never attained, though attainable;—that the average length of human life may be very much extended, and its physical power greatly augmented;—that in every year, within this Commonwealth, thousands of lives are lost which might have been saved;—that tens of thousands of cases of sickness occur, which might have been prevented;—that a vast amount of unnecessarily impaired health, and physical debility exists among those not actually confined by sickness;—that these preventable evils require an enormous expenditure and loss of money, and impose upon the people unnumbered and immeasurable calamities, pecuniary, social, physical, mental, and moral, which might be avoided;—that means exist, within our reach, for their mitigation or removal;—and that measures for prevention will effect infinitely more, than remedies for the cure of disease.* (5, p. 10)

The credo represented a watershed in thinking about health. The resounding optimism reflected in the statement that "perfect health," while seldom achieved, was "attainable" is remarkable in itself. But when Shattuck declares that thousands of lives are needlessly lost, that avoidable sickness exacts a toll that is economic as well as social, physical, mental, and moral, and that prevention creates infinitely more benefit than cure, he is in brave new territory. The ideas constituted a major change in social thought.

The notions, that environmental and social factors are responsible for illness, that the causes of disease can be mitigated or removed, and that prevention rather than remedy is the ultimate solution to health problems, formed the basis of a *sanitary movement*, which had begun in Britain a decade earlier. It had been a turning point. Personal characteristics that had been blamed for disease—lack of cleanliness, intemperance, unemployment, and poverty—were for the first time being seen as *results* rather than *causes* of adverse social and environmental conditions. The polluted water, decaying refuse, open sewers, and airless cellars that had been seen as manifestations of moral disorder began to be appreciated as contributing to, instead of resulting from, human frailty. This new *sanitary science* had been defined as "founded upon a basis of statistical facts...[and] recognizes the invariable and immutable relation subsisting between cause and effect...and projects its measures by rules and laws carefully deduced from a large mass of accurate and reliable observations" (6, p. 209). It fit perfectly with Shattuck's own ideas and sparked the beginning of America's public health movement.

Much of Shattuck's report reflects the influence of British zealots like Edwin Chadwick, with whom Shattuck had corresponded. The overflowing urban centers spawned by the uncontrolled migrations of the industrial revolution had created a sanitary nightmare in Britain of far greater magnitude than anything experienced in America. In *The Sanitary Condition of the Labouring Population of Great Britain*, published in 1842, Chadwick had presented graphic details of the plight of the British working class and the resulting consequences to health. It was this work that codified the sanitary movement and spawned a major shift in attitude—to viewing illness as a collective social ill that was a societal responsibility to remedy. The work made extensive use of sanitary statistics, and Shattuck borrowed freely to illustrate his own report.

Although he referred to his *Sanitary Report* as simply "the outline of a plan" for a survey of the state, it turned out to be much more. Ultimately, the report presented a comprehensive scheme for an entire public health system, including a draft of completely revised public health laws, recommendations to set up boards of health at both the state and local levels, and a host of specific recommendations for creating regulations and gathering data to monitor the ongoing health of the population. There were recommendations regarding building codes, smallpox vaccination requirements, and quarantine of ships; there were recommendations for public bathing houses, for collecting and recycling refuse, for creating institutions for educating females to be nurses, and for making clergymen of all denominations responsible for at least one "discourse" on public health each year. There were 50 recommendations in all.

While many of the brush strokes were broad and visionary, Shattuck offered plenty of details. He specifically suggested, for example, that the state board of health be composed of "two physicians, one councilor of law, one chemist or natural philosopher, one civil engineer, and two persons of other professions or occupations." The physicians, he noted, should "thoroughly understand sanitary science, and deeply feel the importance of wise sanitary measures" (5, pp. 112–113).

One might view the *Report* as approaching the obsessive. Shattuck supplied sample forms for collecting census information, vital statistics, and family health records. And, to be sure that all this advice was presented satisfactorily, he even specified requirements for the resulting publications: "The sanitary and other reports and statements of the affairs of cities and towns which may be printed should be in octavo form, on paper and page of uniform size, and designed to be bound together, as the annual reports of the town" (5, p. 126).

The recommendations were to guide public health policy in the state for years in the future (though not, as it turned out, immediately). It is, however, the first 2 chapters of the report that are most intriguing to our purposes. In these, Shattuck traces the history of the sanitary movement both abroad and in America, giving particular emphasis to the role of vital statistics in identifying health problems. He outlines the history of epidemic diseases in America, beginning in 1618 with an apparent epidemic of yellow fever among the Indians. Proceeding with a chronology of outbreaks of smallpox, typhus, and Asiatic cholera, Shattuck arrives at a vantage point in the middle of the 19th century from which he brandishes his statistics to describe the current state health in Massachusetts.

It is a remarkable work, one that uses data to profile trends in health in a far more sophisticated manner than had been previously seen. His approach to *descriptive statistics*, in which the aggregated characteristics of individuals are elaborated and linked to health outcomes, such as sickness and mortality, form the basis of our present-day approaches. The details are instructive. Shattuck employs several techniques to summarize *mortality* for comparative purposes. Though each technique makes use of the same basic data-deaths in the population—he varies the method of presentation and shows how differences in the way data are depicted can influence our views of health. Table 5-2 illustrates this.

In the table, Shattuck offers data on mortality for three points in time:1830, 1840, and 1845. It is evident that the numbers of deaths in Boston increase. Annual deaths more than double, from 1254 in 1830 to 2903 in 1845. The larger numbers are evident for each age group as well. But how does one interpret these data? Is mortality, in fact, increasing? Is the health of the town declining? Although the growing number of deaths is indisputable, their importance as a health indicator is not. The size of the population from which these deaths arise is also growing. If the number of citizens of Boston is increasing at the same pace as the deaths, there may not be a problem. So a *summary statistic* far more telling than the absolute number of deaths is the number of deaths relative to the number of people in the community. Placing the annual number of deaths for each time period (1254, 1873, 2903) in proportion to the average population at each time (61,392, 85,000, 114,366), we find that the percentage of Bostonians dying each year has grown from 2.0 per 100 to 2.5 per 100–an increase to be sure, but not of the magnitude suggested by the more than twofold rise in numbers of deaths. The increased deaths are more reflective of population growth than of declining health. Proportions such as these (the number of deaths over the number in the population) become *rates* when they are calculated for a particular period of time (for example, one year), and are essential for comparing groups. In a true rate, the people counted in the

TABLE 5-2

Deaths (Number and Percent) by Age Group for Boston in 1830, 1840, and 1845

	1830			1840			1845		
Ages	Annual Deaths	Population	Percent	Annual Deaths	Population	Percent	Annual Deaths	Population	Percent
Under 5	482	8068	6.0	844	11522	7.3	1301	14448	9.0
5 to 15	80	11607	0.7	126	16177	0.8	216	20994	1.0
15 to 30	204	23085	0.9	280	31801	0.9	449	40544	1.1
30 to 50	279	14089	2.0	338	19382	1.7	541	30010	1.8
50 to 70	136	3885	3.5	181	5201	3.5	259	7228	3.6
70 above	74	658	11.2	104	917	11.3	138	1142	12.1
Total	1254	61392	2.0	1873	85000	2.2	2903	114366	2.5

Source: Based on Shattuck (5, p. 82).

TABLE 5-3

Deaths (Number and Percent) by Age Group for Boston and "Country Towns" in 1830

	Boston			Country Towns		
Ages	Deaths	Population	Percent	Deaths	Population	Percent
Under 5	482	8068	6.0	38.2	1249	3.1
5 to 15	80	11607	0.7	9.3	1999	0.5
15 to 30	204	23085	0.9	18.5	2804	0.7
30 to 50	279	14089	2.0	22.1	1881	1.2
50 to 70	136	3885	3.5	20.4	844	2.4
70 above	74	658	11.2	27.5	336	8.2
	1254	61392	2.0	136	9113	1.5

Source: Based on Shattuck (5, p. 82).

numerator are also part of the denominator, since they are alive at some point in the year in which the population estimate is made.*

The *Report* utilizes mortality rates to shed light on the role of *place* in determining health. The relative salubrity of life in the countryside compared with that in urban areas had long been a point of discussion. Regardless of whether one believed the cause was moral or environmental degradation, urban life was widely assumed to be less healthy than rural life. Shattuck now provided evidence that health, at least as measured by mortality, was influenced by where one lived. Table 5-3 compares death by age in Boston with several "country towns" in Massachusetts for 1830.

Two of every 100 residents of Boston die each year compared with only 1.5 per 100 in more rural Massachusetts. The difference is apparent across each age group as well. Almost twice as many children under 5 perish annually in the urban environment than in the outlying towns (6.0% compared with 3.1%). Living in Boston is

---

* The term *rate* is employed casually to describe a variety of proportions—a currency exchange rate, for example. Strictly speaking, these figures are not rates since they lack a relationship to time. Even the "case fatality rate" we discussed with smallpox is not actually a rate, because time is not part of the statistic.

riskier for older folks as well. The annual mortality rate is 11.2%, compared with 8.2% in the country.

Rates are useful for mapping trends but can be hard to conceptualize. Are 2.0 deaths per 100 many or few? Are they more or less than what we should expect? Shattuck employs another mortality statistic that summarizes health status in a way that is easy to understand and can still be used for comparison. He calculates the *average age at death*. This is accomplished by summing the ages of each individual at the time of death and dividing by the total number of deaths that occur. This *average*, also known as a *mean*, presents the middle value of a characteristic of interest-in this case, age. Average age of death is a commonly used comparative health indicator. It is a *summary statistic* that has the advantage of personal salience. Age at death speaks to everyone. Shattuck uses average age at death to dramatize the need for the sanitary survey when he declares "the average age of all that died in Boston, in 1810 to 1820, was 27.85 years, while in 1845, it was 21.43 years only, showing a difference of 6.42 years" (5, p. 104).

While age itself is the most commonly recognized characteristic related to mortality, Shattuck examined others as well. In Table 5-4, he again uses average age at death as his summary

TABLE 5-4

Average Age at Death for Persons in Varying Occupations

Occupations	Avg. Age at Death (yrs.)	Occupations	Avg. Age at Death (yrs.)
Farmers	64.8	Traders	46.8
Coopers	57.4	Cabinet-makers	44.8
Clergymen	56.6	Stone-cutters	44.5
Lawyers	55.5	Shoe-makers	43.4
Physicians	55.0	Laborers	42.8
Blacksmiths	54.5	Seamen	42.5
Carpenters	51.2	Fishermen	41.6
Merchants	50.7	Mechanics	37.2
Masons	48.8	Printers	36.9

Source: Based on Shattuck (5, p. 87).

statistic. This time it is to rank the longevity of workers in a variety of occupations.

There is remarkable variation. Where, on average, farmers may expect to live until almost age 65, mechanics and printers fail to reach even two-score years. Exactly what explains this difference, Shattuck doesn't say. But adding occupation as an attribute deserving of statistical evaluation acknowledges that social and environmental factors may be important determinants of health. Expanding the range of personal characteristics that might influence longevity was a critical contribution of the sanitary movement. Where Rush and Drake limited their consideration of external influences on disease to the atmospheric and topographic, sanitary scientists saw relationships between society, the environment, and the individual as potentially illuminating.

Average age at death is a comprehensible, effective statistic. But Shattuck acknowledges that there can be mischief in the measure:

> The average age at death, as well as the aggregate number of a population out of the whole of which one dies annually, though interesting as a characteristic of the population, is a fallacious test of its sanitary condition; and can not be employed alone for that purpose without leading to serious errors. It can be applied as an accurate test, only when the ages of the living inhabitants compared are alike." (5, pp. 141–142)

He is referring to the fact that the risk of death is not uniformly apportioned through the life span. We know that advancing age carries with it an increased likelihood of death. The occurrence of death among a group of 80-year-olds will be substantially higher than among an equal number of 20-year-olds. But death is also more likely in the first year of life. The period surrounding birth is particularly hazardous. Among communities, distributions of age groups can vary. When they do, comparing averages such as age at death can be misleading. This insight—the recognition that differing *age structures* in populations can influence statistical comparisons—turns out to be one of Shattuck's most profound ones. (Although, again, British colleagues had published on the issue several years earlier.) It creates the basis for one of the most fundamental of principles in the study of disease.

For comparisons to illuminate us on the causes of health outcomes, we must first assume that certain basic characteristics of the populations being compared are similar. We've seen an example with Drake's work on the geography of autumnal fever. Drake assumed that people residing in the various locations he explored had similar risks of acquiring autumnal fever—that they differed only by latitude and climate. However, communities are frequently not at comparable risks for disease or death. The single most important way in which they differ is often with respect to age.

A present-day example may be helpful. Suppose we are in the exploratory stages of retirement planning and are searching for a region of the United States that is a healthy place to spend our golden years. Both Florida (for the warm sun) and Alaska (for its bracing winters) are in contention. Our research uncovers the information in Table 5-5.

Inspecting the table, we discover that the number of deaths occurring in Alaska is far fewer than in Florida. That's not of great surprise, as we reckon the number of people braving life in the far north is considerably lower. To make the comparison meaningful, we need to construct rates that account for the total populations of both states. The third row of the table provides the information we seek. The mortality rate in Florida is more than twice as high as that of Alaska (1062 deaths per 100,000 population compared with 420 deaths per 100,000). That's evidence for a decision.

But before packing up the camper and heading for Alaska, we need one further piece of information. We know that Florida is a popular retirement community. It is likely that there are many more elderly individuals living there than in Alaska. Older folks

TABLE 5-5

Mortality in Florida and Alaska, 1996

	Florida	Alaska
Number of deaths	130,000	3,000
State population	14 million	500 thousand
Mortality rate (deaths/100,000)	1,062	420
Age-adjusted mortality rate (deaths/100,000)	665	663

Source: National Center for Health Statistics (7).

have relatively higher risk for death compared with the younger and more vigorous population that may be attracted to the challenges of living in Alaska. Examination of Figure 5-2 confirms our suspicions. The *age distributions* of people living within the two states are quite different. Over 18% of Floridians are 65 years and over compared with only 5% of Alaskans. This fact can influence the comparison of overall mortality in the two states. Florida has a higher mortality rate, not because it is a less healthy place to live, but because it has an older population. Some sort of "adjustment" that considers the differences in age structure must be made before an adequate comparison can take place. When this is done, the "bottom line" of Table 5-5 shows that the mortality rates are almost identical.

FIGURE 5-2

Distribution of Population by Age, Alaska and Florida, 1996

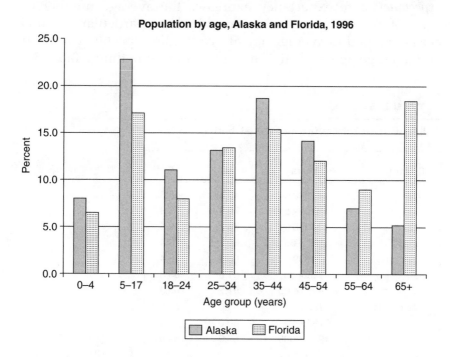

Source: Statistical Abstract of the United States, 1998. (8)

Epidemiologists have several ways of *adjusting for age*. The basic strategy is to compare death rates across the two populations within specific age groups, among 5- to 9-year-olds, 20- to 29-year-olds, and so on. If these *age-specific* rates are comparable, then one can see that the overall mortality experience of each state is similar. Unfortunately, this technique is rather tedious, requiring presentation of a list of age groups and multiple comparative rates. Producing a composite, an *age-adjusted mortality rate,* for each population and then comparing those two numbers can surmount this obstacle. The age-adjusted rate is created by taking age-specific rates for each group and applying them to a large "standard population" (usually that of the entire country) to obtain the numbers of deaths expected for each stratum. These deaths are then summed and divided by the total population to give a summary rate that is *standardized* or *adjusted*. Adjusted rates of groups can be compared without concern that differing age distributions are influencing results.

Another way of presenting mortality data is as *average life expectancy*. Life expectancy expresses the average number of years of life remaining for an individual at a particular age. It is closely related to average age at death. Life expectancy at birth and average age at death amount to the same thing. Table 5-6

TABLE 5-6

Life Expectancy (in Years) at Birth

Country	Years	M	F
USA	1900	46.3	48.3
	1980–85	70.9	78.3
	1998	73.8	79.5
Russia	1980–85	62.1	73.4
	1999	60.0	72.4
Iraq	1980–85	61.5	63.3
	1995–2000	57.2	60.3
South Africa	1980–85	55.0	61.0
	1990–95	60.0	66.0
	1995–2000	53.9	59.6

Sources: National Center for Health Statistics and the United Nations (9, 10, 11).

offers a sample of current life expectancies for some basic characteristics of *person, place,* and *time* around the world. It highlights trends for males and females at different times in different countries. Some rather remarkable information is here. It is evident, for starters, that health in the United States has improved since Shattuck's day. Present-day American males have an average life expectancy at birth of about 74 years, compared with the 46 years of 100 years ago; for American females, the current figure is almost 80 years.

Even trends of the last several decades can be revealing. Most countries have experienced improved conditions and an increasing life expectancy over time. In fact, of the 185 countries listed in the *United Nations' Statistical Yearbook,* 87% enjoyed an increasing life expectancy for both males and females from the period 1980–1985 to 1990–1995 (10). In a handful of countries, however, life expectancy declined. In Russia, and Iraq, both males and females experienced reduced life expectancy. Following the dissolution of the Soviet Union, the new Russia Federation saw social and economic disruption that led to this adverse health. In the aftermath of the Gulf War in 1991 and the consequent international embargoes, average life expectancy in Iraq dropped 4 years for males and 3 years for females. Mortality in South Africa improved following the fall of apartheid only to rise again (decline in life expectancy) with the epidemic of HIV/AIDS.

Another feature of the life expectancy table that merits notice is the almost uniformly higher life span for females than for males. In the United States, women live almost 6 years longer than men, on average. This finding is consistent over time and for most countries and cultures. Even in Shattuck's day, women, on average, outlived men.

Within countries, mortality data can provide insights on the health of subgroups of the population. As Table 5-7 presents the average life expectancy for males and females in the United States, it adds another characteristic of person, race. The dramatic improvements in life expectancy for both sexes and races over the past 100 years are evident—about a 30-year gain for everyone. Again, a persistent advantage is seen for women over their male contemporaries. But the disparity between blacks and whites is also evident. In 1900, black males and females could expect to live an average of only 33

TABLE 5-7

Life Expectancy (in Years) at Birth and at Age 65 by Sex and Race in the United States, 1900, 1980, and 1999

	Male		Female	
	Black	White	Black	White
At birth				
1900	32.5	46.6	33.5	48.7
1980	63.8	70.7	72.5	78.1
1999	67.8	74.6	74.7	79.9
At age 65				
1900	10.4	11.5	11.4	12.2
1980	13.0	14.2	16.8	18.4
1999	14.3	16.1	17.3	19.2

Source: National Center for Health Statistics (9).

years; their white contemporaries averaged almost 15 years more. In 1998, there is still a discrepancy, though the difference has narrowed considerably. The life expectancy of a white male child at birth is about 75 years compared with 68 for a black male; at birth, white females can now anticipate to live until 80, about 5 more years than a black female.

However, life expectancy at birth tells only a part of the story. The lower half of Table 5-7 displays the life expectancy, the average years of life remaining, for individuals who have already attained the age of 65. Note that the improvements between 1900 and 1998 are much less striking. In 1900, an average 65-year-old could anticipate from 10 to 12 additional years of life. A century later the figures have increased by only 4 to 7 years. And, although differences are evident between the races and sexes, they are less dramatic than differences at birth. (Of course, by the time we reach the 7th decade of life, the opportunity for improvement becomes somewhat limited.)

A major factor affecting life expectancy is the vulnerable period occurring during the first years of life, as Shattuck recognized. The death rate is higher in the year following birth than at any time during the life span until the age of 65. It contributes substantially to the calculations of average age at death when there are large numbers of infants in the population. In fact, *infant mortality* has become a widely used indicator of health in its own right. Table 5-8 adds infant mortality to the life expectancy data we've just seen. The table shows that for the United States, a substantial drop in the infant mortality rate accompanies the increase in life expectancy. At present, infant mortality is at its lowest point ever. Countries that lead the world with even lower rates are Japan and a number of northern European nations.

Unfortunately, in much of the developing world, infant mortality is as high at the close of the 20th century as it was in 19th-century America. Look closely at Table 5-8. The changes in infant mortality from the early 1980s to the 1990s among countries where the life expectancy fell are revealing. In Iraq, for example, one is not surprised to see the infant mortality rate rising during the time the country was punished by international embargoes. Infants and children suffered greatly. In Russia, on the other hand, infant mortality actually declined during the period of social and political upheaval. The cause of Russia's drop in average years of life cannot be attributed to its infant mortality. It is due to increased mortality among

TABLE 5-8

Life Expectancy (in Years) at Birth, and Infant Mortality (Deaths/1000 Live Births)

Country Mortality	Years	M	F	Infan
USA	1900	46.3	48.3	100
	1980–85	70.9	78.3	11
	1998	73.8	79.5	7
Russia	1980–85	62.1	73.4	26
	1995	58.3	71.7	18
	1999	60.0	72.4	17
Iraq	1980–85	61.5	63.3	78
	1995–2000	57.2	60.3	92
South Africa	1980–85	55.0	61.0	63
	1990–95	60.0	66.0	53
	1995–2000	53.9	59.6	58

young and middle-aged adults and can be linked to rising rates of injuries from automobiles and guns. Most are alcohol related. The rapid social changes that followed the collapse of the Communist state had profound health consequences. The table suggests some improvement in more recent years.

In the United States, infant mortality has been a source of concern for years. Table 5-9 demonstrates that infant mortality for blacks has always been about twice as high as that for whites. Even though the rates for blacks have come down sharply, they remain disproportionately high—an indicator of a national health problem.

Infant mortality, like overall mortality, is expressed as a *rate*—the number of deaths in the population that occur over a period of one year. But the denominator differs from the one used to express general mortality. In this instance, deaths are reported for every 1000 live births, not the number of persons in the community. Why the change? Once more, the need is to find a denominator that creates appropriate comparisons. Comparing infant mortality in Alaska and Florida would fall prey to the same age distribution differences we saw before. Death rates based on the entire Florida population might appear lower, not because of better health outcomes but because the state has a smaller proportion of women giving birth.

Shattuck recognized that the differential mortality rates he observed across communities in Massachusetts had implications beyond fueling the debate on the evils of city living. The lower mortality rates of the "country towns" were proof that better health was possible. The mortality of cities was excessive:

TABLE 5-9

Infant Mortality by Race, 1960, 1980 and 1999 (Deaths per 1000 Live Births)

	Black	White
1960	44.3	22.9
1980	22.2	10.9
1999	14.6	5.8

Source: National Center for Health Statistics (9).

> In Boston, during thirty-nine years, 1811 to 1849 inclusive, 62,431 deaths took place, of which 2,079, or 3.33 per cent only, were from old age, and 96.67 per cent from diseases and other causes.... Is it not a practical measure to prevent some of this great amount of disease, and assist some of these lives that they may grow old, and die only because they are old?" (5, p. 244)

This reasoning leads him to an interesting calculation. Applying the healthier, 1.5 percent death rate found in the country towns to the Boston population, Shattuck reckons that, typically, over 1100 unnecessary deaths occur on an annual basis. Extrapolating the calculation to the state as a whole, he decides that as many as 6000 unnecessary deaths occur each year. In addition to the personal grief and suffering such loss of life engenders, Shattuck adds another consideration:

> The number of unnecessary deaths the past year, has been estimated at 6,000.... This is a direct pecuniary loss to the State. If each of these 6,000 had been saved, and had lived 18 years, which may be taken as the average length of the labor-period of life; or if the whole 18,000 persons who died in the State, could have lived, on the average, six years longer than they did, (and who will they say that they might not more than that period?) then we have 108,000 years of lost labor on their account which may fairly be estimated at $50 each per annum.... Then there are the public paupers, widows and orphans, made so by the premature deaths of relatives, which cannot be estimated at less than 6,000 at $1 per week. According to this calculation we have—
>
> Loss of 108,000 years of labor, at $50 per annum, $5,400,000
>
> Cost of supporting 6,000 widows and orphans, at $52 per annum, $312,000. (5)

An economic dimension has been added to the problems of poor health and early death. It suggests another way of expressing mortality, as premature death, or *years of potential life lost*. Years of potential life lost (YPLL) is a concept in use today. Its value lies in distinguishing the impact of diseases that take their toll in life's later years from those where there is a greater burden on the young. Table 5-10 shows recent data comparing several causes of death by their overall mortality rates and years of potential life lost. Note that the *anticipated* length of life is 75 years.

Over 4 times as many people die from heart disease each year as from unintentional injuries. Yet the years of potential life lost are almost the same for the 2 causes of death. Rates of death due to diabetes are comparable to those of motor vehicle-associated injury deaths (14 per hundred thousand and 16 per hundred thousand,

TABLE 5-10

Death Rate and Years of Potential Life Lost (YPLL) for
Selected Conditions, United States, 1996 (per 100,000
Population)

Condition	Death Rate	YPLL
Heart disease	135	1223
Cancer	128	1554
Diabetes	14	154
Unintentional injuries	30	1137
Motor vehicle–related injuries	16	681
HIV* infection	11	402

*Human immunodeficiency virus
Source: National Center for Health Statistics (9).

respectively). But the motor vehicle-related fatalities create almost 4
times the loss of potential life years. Deaths related to infection with
HIV are down the list on the death rate rankings, only 11 per hundred thousand. But the disease assumes much greater importance
when YPLL are considered (402 per hundred thousand). The reason
for the apparent "discrepancy" is evident. Unintentional injuries,
motor vehicle-related injuries, and deaths due to HIV infection strike
younger individuals on average than do heart disease, cancer, and
diabetes.

Examine the sequential tables that compare mortality from
unintentional injuries (excluding causes such as homicide and sui-
cide) for the two age groups, 15 through 24 years and 65 years and
over, for the 2 years 1980 and 1998.

Table 5-11a shows simply the total number of deaths for each
category. The trends for the two age groups are strikingly different.
There has been a 50% drop in injury deaths for the younger ages
(26,000 deaths down to 13,000) and a substantial increase for the
older group (24,000, rising to almost 33,000). What is the explanation? Is it becoming more hazardous in our society for older folks
and safer for the younger ones? A first thought should be that
perhaps the denominators, the population at risk, has changed
for the two groups (though it is worth noting that a substantial

TABLE 5-11

Mortality from Unintentional Injury for Age Groups 15 to 24 Years and 65 Years and Over, United States, 1980 and 1998

a. Total Deaths

	1980	1998
15 to 24 years	26,206	13,349
65 years and over	24,844	32,975

b. Death Rate per 100,000

	1980	1998
15 to 24 years	75.1 (26,206 per 34.9 million)	35.9 (13,349 per 37.3 million)
65 years and over	97.4 (24,844 per 25.5 million)	95.9 (32,975 per 34.4 million)

c. Proportionate Mortality (Percent)

	1980	1998
15-24 years	53.5 (26,206/49,027)	43.6 (13,349/30,627)
65 years and over	1.9 (24,844/1,341,848)	1.9 (32,975/1,753,220)

Source: National Center for Health Statistics (9).

population shift would be required to affect such a change). Sure enough, when the denominators (the total population in each particular age group) is included, the story changes. As seen in Table 5-11*b*, when rates per 100,000 population are examined, mortality for the 15- through 24-year-olds has, indeed, dropped to about half the level in 1998 as in 1980. But for those 65 years and over, there has been no such improvement. Rates have remained almost unchanged over the 18 years. The 33% increase in deaths among older individuals reflects, not growing danger, but an increasingly older population. The number of 15- to 24-year-olds has grown as well. But the decline in injury deaths in the group persists after the population change is factored in, serving as another reminder of the importance of using the appropriate population at risk (in this case, an age-specific group) when making comparisons.

One additional way of looking at these mortality figures gives a slightly different slant. Table 5-11c shows mortality from unintentional injuries as a proportion of the total deaths for each age group. This presentation of *proportionate mortality* shows the importance of a particular cause of death in relation to other causes within the age group. Shattuck used the concept of proportionate mortality when he showed the increasing proportions of total mortality among children less than 5 years of age. The table shows that injuries are a very substantial cause of death for younger individuals. In contrast among the older age group, injury deaths, although numerous, account for only 2% of the total. Although the injury rate among the 65 and overs in 1998 is almost 3 times that of the younger group, its relative importance as a cause of death is small.

Each of these presentations of mortality offers a slightly different perspective on the problem. If one asks, "what is the importance of injury deaths in the two age groups," the response depends on how you think about the data. More people die from unintentional injury in the older group, and the rate is higher. But with many competing causes of mortality after the age of 65, the proportionate impact is less. If one were planning health interventions targeted at specific ages and wanted to maximize effectiveness, the way one looked at the data could influence resource allocation.

The *Shattuck Report* was well received when it appeared in January 1851. Letters of appreciation came from as far as Josiah Nott in Mobile, Alabama, and the English government offices in Whitehall. The Philadelphia Board of Health passed a resolution praising the "very comprehensive and valuable report" (12), and editorialists in the Boston and New York medical and surgical journals reviewed it favorably. One colleague, Dr. Stephen West Williams, of Deerfield, Massachusetts, was so impressed that he immediately volunteered to serve on Shattuck's proposed state board of health. "I think it [the report] the most able document by far which I have ever seen in any language," wrote Williams. "If it [the proposal for the board] passes I should like to be a member of the Board of Health" (12).

In support of his qualifications for the post, Williams offers his publication on the climate and diseases of his native Deerfield (in the western Connecticut Valley region of Massachusetts), in which he records his own discovery of the benefits of country living. (13) He finds that Deerfield has a mortality rate only three-quarters that of Boston and proudly concludes that "a healthier locality can not be found on the surface of the globe than Deerfield" (13).

Although Dr. Williams shared Shattuck's hopes that the Massachusetts General Court would embrace the *Report*'s ideas, noting that "Massachusetts has always been a pioneer in such undertakings," the legislature accepted it, but did nothing else. None of the 50 recommendations that Shattuck so painstakingly produced saw implementation. The extensive catalog of plans for organizing, regulating, educating, and monitoring to improve the health of citizens of the Commonwealth was relegated to the shelves of the General Court. Not until almost 20 years had passed and Shattuck had been dead for a decade, was the principle recommendation taken up and a State Board of Health created.

Following the flurry that accompanied publication, Shattuck quietly returned to the genealogy he loved. In 1855 he published a 400-page tome that traced seven generations of Shattucks back to the 17th century (14). In it he details the births, marriages, and deaths of 4121 of his American ancestors, punctuating the vital records with personal comments. True to his nature, he cannot resist applying statistical tools to his own family's story. He finds, for example, that the ratio of male-to-female births was 109:100 and that 72 sets of twins had been produced ("or 1 in every 57th child born"). Included are calculations on the average age of marriage of successive generations, the average duration of married life, and the interval between first and second marriages. He even computes, with characteristic precision, the average age of death for his ancestors—53 years, 6 months, 8 days, with a difference between the males and females of only 8 months, 16 days in favor of the women. The "average age (of death) of all the males who survived 20 years," he finds, "was 63 years, 5 months, 1 day" (14).

When Shattuck compares this figure to the numbers for all Massachusetts professions (51 years, 7 months, 28 days), a hint of unstatistical chauvinism creeps in: "The law of mortality, thus ascertained to exist in our family, is more favorable to a strong vital force and to longevity than in the average of mankind" (14).

It might have been true. Certainly, Shattuck himself was not an average man.

REFERENCES

1. Shattuck L. *History of the Town of Concord, Middlesex County, Massachusetts.* Concord: John Stacy; 1835.
2. Shattuck L. *The Vital Statistics of Boston; Containing an Abstract of the Bills of Mortality for the Last Twenty-nine Years, and a General View of the Population and Health of the City at Other Periods of Its History.* Philadelphia: Lea & Blanchard; 1841.
3. Willcox WF. Lemuel Shattuck: statist, founder of the American Statistical Association. *J Amer Statistical Assoc.* 1940; 35:224–235.
4. Rosenkrantz BG. *Public Health and the State-Changing Views in Massachusetts, 1842–1936:* Harvard University Press; 1972.
5. Shattuck L. *Report of the Sanitary Commission of Massachusetts 1850.* Cambridge: Harvard University Press; 1948.
6. Cassedy JH. *American Medicine and Statistical Thinking, 1800–1860.* Cambridge: Harvard University Press; 1984.
7. *Health, United States, 2000.* Hyattsville, MD: National Center for Health Statistics; 2000.
8. U.S. Bureau of the Census. *Statistical Abstract of the United States: 1998 (118th edition).* Washington, DC; 1998.
9. *Health, United States, 2002.* Hyattsville, MD: National Center for Health Statistics; 2002.
10. Department of Economic and Social Affairs Statistics Division. Health and child-bearing. *Statistical Yearbook, Forty-Second Issue, 1995.* New York: United Nations; 1997:79–85.
11. Department of Economic and Social Affairs. *1996 Demographic Yearbook.* Vol. 48. New York: United Nations; 1998:762.

12. Shattuck L. *Lemuel Shattuck Papers, 1805–1867*. Boston: Massachusetts Historical Society;

13. Williams S. Medical and physical topography of the town of Deerfield, Franklin Co., Massachusetts. Boston *Med Surg J*. 1836; 15:197–202.

14. Shattuck L. *Memorials of the Descendents of William Shattuck the Progenitor of the Families in America that Have Borne His Name; Including an Introduction, and an Appendix Containing Collateral Information*. Boston: Dutton & Wentworth; 1855.

CHAPTER 6

Adirondack Cure: Consumption and Edward Trudeau

He was struck with death about two o'clock in the afternoon at which time the bed on which he lay shook—so violent were the convulsions of dissolving nature. Twelve with myself spent the night, watching round the bed of this beloved man. He sometimes opened his eyes, and looked on his dear family. Although unable to speak his countenance expressed the greatness of his affection. About 11 he revived a little. My stepmother, standing by him, took his hand—he excited all his dying efforts, and, looking upon her with inexpressible tenderness, closed her hand in his....He lay in great distress during the whole night—now and then a deep sigh, accompanied by a feeble groan, escaped him, while obstructing phlegm continually rattled with every breath. He retained his reason so long as he had strength to manifest it....The sweat poured with such freedom as to wet the sheets and even the bed itself. The morning came. A serene stillness reigned throughout all nature—no cloud obscured the sky, but all was calm and pleasant....The sun had just illumined our world with his bright beams and shown into the apartment with peculiar luster, where lay the dying saint, about to abandon forever his clay tenements and (I think) enter that blessed region, where they have no need of the sun for Jesus, the Lamb of God is the light thereof. In a few moments he turned his eyes upwards, as though he viewed the indescribable glories of the upper world-his mouth closed, and a few feeble gasps released his labouring soul from the prison of flesh, and I have much reason to believe entered himself into the joy of his Lord. (1)

Lemuel Shattuck's father died on April 27, 1816, at the age (recorded with Shattuck's characteristic precision) of 58 years, 9 months, and 20 days. The poignant words describing his final hours were set down by Shattuck's sister Rebecca. It is a melancholy piece that, with variations, was played over and over throughout the 19th century. John Shattuck had succumbed to a lingering struggle with consumption. According to the younger Shattuck, his father had caught cold the previous September while visiting relatives. This had "settled upon his lungs and fixed and accelerated a disease from which he never recovered" (1). The labored respirations, obstructing phlegm, and drenching sweats were characteristic of the disease. Consumption was aptly named. Unlike the rapidly acting, decisive diseases like smallpox and yellow fever, consumption came on gradually, beginning as an apparently inconsequential respiratory infection (a "cold") that lingered on, as persistent fevers, disquieting sweats, and a seeming dissolution of the body. Victims were indeed "consumed;" the appetite declined, weight disappeared, and the skin took on a pale, almost transparent appearance. As the disease progressed, there were incapacitating paroxysms of coughing. These turned most ominous when the resulting phlegm became first tinged with blood and then bright red with it.

Consumption is another disease with origins in antiquity. The Greeks had called it *phthisis*, which means to waste away, and the illness had long been recognized as a protracted struggle that could go on for months or even years. Occasionally, there were remissions in which the incessant, incapacitating cough might relent, the appetite improve somewhat, and the persistent fevers abate. But symptoms would return and, it was widely acknowledged, the decline to death was inevitable.

Shattuck had devoted considerable space to consumption in the *Report of the Sanitary Commission of Massachusetts 1850* (2). Of the 10 pages allotted to detailed accounts of diseases that influence the sanitary condition of the state, 6 were given to consumption. There was good reason. Of the 57,000 deaths recorded in Massachusetts between 1842 and 1848, almost 24% were from consumption. It was the largest single cause of death, by a factor of more than 2. Shattuck notes "that great destroyer of human health and human life...the first rank...agent of death...takes its subjects principally at the productive period of life, 15–60, the precious and most useful season. In the ages 20–30, 'the beauty and hope of life,'—far more die than at other ages." Young women who resided in the Massachusetts countryside were particularly susceptible, perishing in twice the numbers as men. In cities, the reverse was true; deaths were greater among males. Consumption, Shattuck lamented, "is a constant visitor in all parts of our Commonwealth—on the mountains of Berkshire and the valley of the Connecticut as well as along the seacoast." It perplexed him that, while *epidemic* diseases created alarm and prompted precautionary measures for prevention, consumption did not. He wondered, "where is the alarm and caution against a more inexorable disease, which in this state, in everyday and every year deprives more than 7 human beings of their lives?" (2, pp. 94–98). The fact was, consumption was so pervasive in the middle and late 19th century that it had become an accepted burden of existence.

As with the other diseases we have examined, the cause of consumption was contested but unknown. There were the usual speculations about miasmas and suspicions about climate, which were not surprising, given the observations that cold, damp environments appeared to harbor greater numbers of consumptives. A stubborn few people considered contagion a possibility, but they carried little credibility. The dominant view was that consumption was hereditary—it ran in families. There was ample evidence in support of this belief. Shattuck's own family was a convincing example. Eighteen years before his father's death, Shattuck lost his mother to the disease. She was, he records, "not blessed naturally, with a strong constitution. There appeared lurking in her system some hereditary tendency to consumption the disease from which she died. Her mother and one of her sisters, though surviving her, died of that disease" (1). While Shattuck himself escaped its depredations, his sister, Rebecca, who wrote the moving description of their father's death, succumbed to the disease only 1 year later.

The Shattucks were far from the only family in which consumption "ran." Many others, some quite notable, shared the constitutional affliction. The family of Ralph Waldo Emerson, a Concord neighbor of the Shattucks, was also burdened with consumption. Ralph Waldo's father, the Reverend William Emerson, died of the disease, as did 3 of Emerson's brothers. Older brother John was only 6 when he succumbed. Another brother, Edward, died at 29, and Charles Chauncey Emerson, the youngest, was embarking on a promising legal career when he perished at the age of 27. Though Emerson's oldest surviving brother, William, was never diagnosed as phthistical, he did hire a neighbor from another family with a long history of consumption as a tutor for his 7-year-old son. Henry Thoreau worked for the Emersons briefly before he took up residence at Walden Pond. Twenty years later, Thoreau died of the disease.

Perhaps the saddest episode in the Emerson saga was the story of Ralph Waldo's young bride, Ellen Tucker. Ellen was only 16 when Emerson courted her, but she was already perishing of the disease. Emerson married Ellen Tucker knowing her condition—aware that she was unlikely to survive much past her wedding—which, indeed, she did not. Ellen embodied the early 19th-century view of the consumptive: a delicate young woman with pale almost translucent skin; a detached, almost otherworldly quality, chaste in her brief, faultless life. This was the romantic age, and consumption was imbued with mystical, almost desirable, qualities.

Romanticized characterizations were prevalent in stories of the time. Concord's most famous fictional family, the March family from *Little Women*, was also tragically beset:

> When Jo came home that spring, she had been struck with the change in Beth. No one spoke of it or seemed aware of it, for it had come too gradually to startle those who saw her daily; but to eyes sharpened by absence it was very plain, and a heavy weight fell on Jo's heart as she saw her sister's face. It was no paler, and but little thinner than in autumn; yet there was a strange transparent look about it, as if the mortal was being slowly refined away, and the immortal shining through the frail flesh with an indescribably pathetic beauty. (3, p. 24)

Another family in which consumption was to play a pivotal role was that of Edward Livingston Trudeau. The Trudeau family roots extended back to 18th-century Louisiana soil, where, in 1794, an enterprising lieutenant governor named Zenon Trudeau organized an expedition to explore the upper reaches of the Missouri River. The adventure was to founder, but portions of a journal of the trip, which detailed the routes taken and Indian tribes encountered, found their way to Thomas Jefferson and ultimately assisted Captain Merriweather Lewis and his Corps of Discovery. Zenon's grandson, James Trudeau, was the family's first physician, but neglected his practice to pursue his passion for the outdoor life. James spent more time on outings with his friend, John J. Audubon, sketching and preparing ornithological specimens than he did aiding his patients.

The wanderlust that undid James's medical practice undermined his marriage as well. In 1848, a few months after the birth of his 3rd child, Edward, James abandoned his family, prompting his wife to seek lodging with her father, also a physician, in Paris. Edward, who becomes the focus of our story, spent his childhood in France, returning to America with his brother as a teenager to settle with New York relations.

As a young man, Edward embarked on a nautical career, enrolling in a preparatory school in Newport, Rhode Island, en route to the Naval Academy. His plans changed abruptly however, when he was called back to New York to attend his critically ill older brother. Francis, it was apparent, was dying of consumption.

As was the custom, Trudeau became his brother's nurse, filling the vacuum of effective medical care with the comfort of companionship. Years later, Trudeau recalled:

> We occupied the same room and sometimes the same bed. I bathed him and brought his meals to him, and when he felt well enough to go downstairs I carried him up and down on my back, and I tried to amuse and cheer him through the long days of fever and sickness. My sister and grandmother often sat with him in the daytime and allowed me to go out for exercise and change, but he soon became very dependent upon me and I had to be with him day and night. The doctor called once a week to see him and usually left some new cough medicine, but the cough grew steadily worse. Not only did the doctor never advise any precautions to protect me against infection, but he told me repeatedly never to open the windows, as it would aggravate the cough; and I never did, until toward the end my brother was so short of breath that he asked for fresh air. (4, p. 30)

The efforts were unsuccessful. Francis succumbed two days before Christmas in 1867:

> It was my first great sorrow. It nearly broke my heart, and I have never ceased to feel its influence. In after years it developed in me an unquenchable sympathy for all (consumption) patients—a sympathy which I hope has grown no less through a lifetime spent in trying to express it practically. Even now I love to think that my work has been in a measure a tribute from me to the brother I loved so well. (4, p. 31)

After his brother died, Trudeau drifted. He made several attempts to find a vocation, spending 3 months as a student in a School

of Mines and then trying out the brokerage business. In the autumn
of 1868, on an impulse he later described as an "auto-suggestion,
perhaps imparted by the blood of [his] ancestors" (4, p. 37), he
enrolled in New York's College of Physicians and Surgeons. His
friends thought it an improbable impulse. One fellow member of
New York's Union Club, where Trudeau and his friends idled
many hours, offered a bet of 500 dollars that Trudeau would never
graduate. Undeterred by such skepticism, Edward went forward
with the plan and soon was rapt in his studies.

Not surprisingly, the subject of most interest to the fledgling
doctor was consumption. From Dr. Alonzo Clark, Trudeau learned
that consumption was "a non contagious, generally incurable and
inherited disease due to inherited peculiarities, perverted humors,
and various types of inflammation" (4, p. 40). Trudeau mastered
what was known about the pathology of the disease—the abnormal
properties of the afflicted lungs. Several findings had become well
documented. When examined, the consumptive lung showed invasion by small firm nodules, or *tubercles*, that displaced and destroyed
healthy, functioning tissue. Under the increasing scrutiny of
European microscopes, these nodules appeared as small pockets—
rings of cells with cheesy, noncellular centers. It was apparent that
the substance within the tubercles was the residue of destroyed
cells, the aftermath of fierce, unseen battles. Medical science was
advancing; its descriptive power was growing, becoming more
detailed and precise. Reference to the disease itself was also becoming more scientific. The nonspecific label of *consumption*, the wasting disease, was increasingly being replaced with the pathologic
designation, *tuberculosis*.

Trudeau completed his medical studies, including a 3-year
attachment to the practice of a local physician and a 6-month post
in New York's Strangers Hospital. They were active, heady years.
Trudeau had inherited (in addition to his medical calling) a love of
the outdoors. He was an avid walker, horseman, hunter, and
oarsman, often rowing great stretches of the Hudson River, from
Rhinebeck to Manhattan. Challenged by comrades to prove his fit-
ness, he walked from Central Park to the Battery at the tip of the
island in just 47 minutes (4, pp. 50–51).

At the completion of his training, Trudeau married a Long
Island rector's daughter and struggled with a country practice on

Little Neck, Long Island. But finding it "monotonous," he moved back to New York City. All this time there were growing hints of problems with his health:

> While at Little Neck I had on two or three occasions attacks of fever, but as nearly everybody had malaria I was told it was malaria and took quinine which, however, did little good. After we moved into town I felt tired all the time, but thought it was the confinement of the city life and paid but little attention to it. (4, p. 70)

Finally, he yielded to a colleague's prodding and submitted to a physical examination. The upper two-thirds of his left lung was being consumed by active tuberculosis. Trudeau was devastated:

> I think I know something of the feelings of the man at the bar who is told he is to be hanged on a given date, for in those days pulmonary consumption was considered as absolutely fatal. I pulled myself together, put as good a face on the matter as I could, and escaped from the office after thanking the doctor for his examination. When I got outside, as I stood on [the doctor's] stoop, I felt stunned. It seemed to me the world had suddenly grown dark. The sun was shining, it is true, and the street was filled with the rush and noise of traffic, but to me the world had lost every vestige of brightness. I had consumption—that most fatal of diseases! (4, p. 71)

Faced with a grim and limited future, Trudeau fled. If his days were numbered, he did not want to spend them in New York City. By May 1873, only a few months after the fatal diagnosis was pronounced, he was on a train heading north up the Hudson River. After a difficult 5-day journey that concluded with a jolting, 42-mile wagon ride over a corduroy road, he arrived at Paul Smith's rustic hotel on St. Regis Lake in the heart of the Adirondack Mountains. He was exhausted. So depleted was this shell of a once-rugged outdoorsman that he had to be carried to his room in the arms of Smith's brother-in-law.

When some strength was returned, Trudeau began to venture out. His first excursions were limited to rowboat trips, in which he would lie on blankets on the bottom of a boat while a staff member toured him around the lake. Over the summer, he improved. His cough diminished. The fever abated. By the autumn, he had gained 15 pounds and was ready to return to his wife and two young children in New York City (see Figure 6-1). It was a miracle. Trudeau had not expected remedy. He had traveled to the Adirondacks

FIGURE 6-1

Edward Trudeau After His First Summer in the Adirondacks

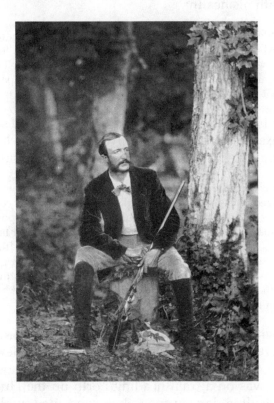

Source: Trudeau Institute Archives.

intending his departure from the world. Now, thanks to the fresh forest air, rest, and good nutrition, he was rejoining it.

His marvelous recovery was, however, not sustained. Soon after his return to New York, Trudeau relapsed. His doctors suggested that he winter in St. Paul, Minnesota, a place recommended for "pulmonary invalids" because of its large number of sunny days. It was not a success. Trudeau was feverish for most of the winter and by spring was as sick as he had been the year before. In June he returned to the Adirondacks, this time accompanied by his family. Progress was not as dramatic as the previous summer.

Trudeau and his wife made the bold decision that the family should remain in the Adirondacks.

Winters in this upper reach of New York State were not for the faint of heart. No outside visitors had ever wintered there before. This was a place entirely cut off from the outside world, 60 miles from the nearest doctor or railroad. Indeed, the season provided arduous moments, but the family survived and Trudeau's condition stabilized.

He was now committed to the Adirondacks, convinced that the prescription of fresh air, rest, and diet was the key to defeating tuberculosis. In the years that followed, he continued to experience exacerbations of his disease. But the illness was sufficiently controlled that he began to think of practicing medicine again. He also vowed to share his epiphany of cure with other tuberculosis sufferers. The family settled at Saranac Lake, in a tiny village where, for $25 a month, the Trudeaus rented a small clapboard house owned by one of the local guides. There, he began to make plans for a treatment facility that was to become the "now famous health resort known as Saranac Lake" (4, p. 123).

Trudeau was not the first to come upon the notion of fresh air and rest to treat tuberculosis. Consumptive patients had been seeking beneficial climates for some years. Opinions on the places best suited to such purposes varied. Some doctors favored locations that were warm and dry; others preferred the cold and bracing; still others recommended the heat and humidity of the tropics. For many years, consumptive young men were prescribed voyages at sea where the fresh salt air and gently rolling waves were thought to be therapeutic. Some doctors even suggested that "occasional vomiting, which persons unaccustomed to be on board of a ship usually experience," was part of the treatment (5, p. 19).

Overland travel was also a popular recommendation. The idea that the activity of the travel itself was beneficial was a holdover from 17th-century England, where the famous physician Thomas Sydenham had enthusiastically endorsed horseback riding as a potent remedy for consumption. Several New England doctors also promoted this approach. Boston's Dr. Bowditch, for example, reported that his father had been cured of consumption by a 748-mile journey through New England, in an open *chaise* (5, p. 20).

The American west was a particularly popular destination, in part for its warm, dry climate, but also for the strenuous overland trip that was required. Daniel Drake recommended several "journeys of health on the great plains" in which invalids might, "in the voiceless solitudes of the desert...pitch their tents and plunge into rustication." The route to Santa Fe offered "the luscious vineyards of the El Paso...the rich and beautiful valley of Taos," and "snowy summits (that) refresh with cool and strength-giving breezes." Health benefits accrued from "the drier air, hard bed, simple diet, saddle exercise, divestiture of cares, and redemption from the dominion of empiricism and polypharmacy". Conceding that "these journeys abound in exposures, fatigues and privations," Drake advised that, "it is on them that the benefit chiefly depends. Take them away, and a journey over the desert to the Rocky Mountains would be scarcely more efficacious than the fashionable voyage to Europe." Among the conditions most amenable to journey cures was "tubercular consumption in every stage, from earliest predisposition to that in which the patient has merely the ability to keep in his saddle through the day" (6, pp. 174–175).

Credit for creation of the first organized health retreat for tuberculous patients goes to a German named Hermann Brehmer, who created a sanatorium* in Europe's Silesian Mountains in 1854. Brehmer, like Trudeau, had come across the idea of climate as cure from personal experience. His own case of tuberculosis had improved in the cold, pure air of the Himalayas. By the 1870s, other Europeans had followed Brehmer's lead and more sanatoria were opened to provide rest, fresh air, and strict regulation of the patient's life and habits (see Figure 6-2). Trudeau would become the first in America to develop a retreat dedicated not only to the care of consumptives but to the scientific pursuit of curing tuberculosis.

---

* The two terms *sanitarium* and *sanatorium* are often used interchangeably to describe tuberculosis retreats. The roots of the words and their meanings differ slightly. Sanitarium comes from *sanitas*, meaning "health," and suggests a healthy environment or health resort. Sanatorium comes from *sanare*, which means "to heal or cure" and suggests the remedial or restorative intent. Trudeau originally created the Adirondack Cottage Sanitarium, which became the Trudeau Sanatorium following his death—a tribute not only to the man but to the potency of his methods.

FIGURE 6-2

The Winter Cure for Tuberculosis

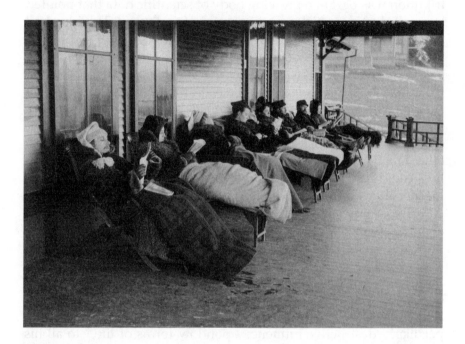

Source: Trudeau Institute Archives.

This second, more ambitious element of his plan was novel. Prior to the spring of 1882 Trudeau would not have considered himself a medical researcher. He had no background in research, nor any demonstrated interest. But in March 1882 an event occurred that changed him entirely. That month at a Berlin scientific meeting, a 39-year-old German doctor read a paper in which he announced the discovery of the cause of tuberculosis. Robert Koch's paper astonished the world. Here was the solution to the puzzle that had plagued humankind for so many generations. According to Koch, the element responsible for the monumental suffering of millions of people over dozens of centuries was a single microscopic cell. It was a living organism capable of multiplying in the human body. And it was contagious—transmitted from person to person.

The tuberculosis bacillus was not Koch's first microbiologic discovery. Six years earlier, in 1876, he had identified the source of a disease that had plagued livestock since antiquity, isolating and cultivating the microorganism responsible for anthrax. Koch's contribution was part of a growing body of scientific data that pointed to small, living particles as responsible for disease. The idea had surfaced periodically for many years, only to be dismissed by the theoreticians on each occasion. Cotton Mather had suggested it, as had Daniel Drake. In 1865, evidence that tuberculosis might be contagious had been presented by a French army surgeon named Jean-Antoine Villemin. Villemin injected material from tubercles from a human dead of tuberculosis into rabbits. The rabbits developed their own tubercles. He then used the material from the rabbits to infect other rabbits and guinea pigs. His experiments showed that tuberculosis could be transmitted, and whatever "principle" was present in the inoculums he used multiplied after it was injected.

Two years later a British surgeon named Joseph Lister made another discovery. Like many others, Lister was dismayed by high rates of suppuration and putrefaction (infection) that occurred among patients who had open wounds. He decided that unseen, airborne particles were responsible. To counteract these infecting agents, Lister devised a system he called *antisepsis*. He began applying carbolic acid, "a volatile organic compound, which appears to exercise a peculiarly destructive influence upon low forms of life," to all his patients' wounds. Infection rates plummeted (7). Using an entirely different approach, Lister had reinforced Villeman's findings that living, invisible particles could transmit disease and that this transmission might be prevented.

The evidence from Europe was tilting increasingly in the direction of microbes as causal agents. In addition to Villemin and Lister, there was the brilliant Louis Pasteur, Lister's source of inspiration. It was Pasteur who had first demonstrated that particles invisible to the human eye were abroad in the atmosphere and capable of spoiling wine, infecting silk worms, and likely, causing human wounds to fester. Several fungi had been identified and linked to animal diseases. In 1878 Koch reported linking 6 different types of surgical infections to 6 specific bacteria.

But many people needed more convincing proof. Belief that diseases were the result of intrinsic human failings (albeit exacerbated by unfavorable environments) still ran strong. The microbes that were being increasingly observed in disease states could be a *consequence* rather than a *cause* of disease. That specific germs might be responsible for particular diseases flew against many cherished beliefs. One outspoken critic noted "the specific disease doctrine is the grand refuge of weak, uncultured, unstable minds, such as now rule in the medical profession" (8, p. 249). That vocal critic, Florence Nightingale, was a woman not easily influenced by the evidence of others. Another critic disparaged the experiments that demonstrated disease transmissibility in rabbits, arguing that the evidence was not convincing because "the rabbit is a melancholy animal to whom life is a burden and who only asks to leave it" (8, p. 243).

What Koch added to the debate was a clear head and almost flawless experimental technique. He was able to solve laboratory problems that had stymied those before him. By meticulous persistence, he devised a method for staining the tuberculosis germ so that it was visible in tissues examined under the microscope. He was also able to propagate the bacterium in laboratory culture media once he recognized that the germ grew much more slowly than anticipated. Finally, he set out rules for determining when an agent was, in fact, the cause of a disease. These became known as *Koch's postulates* and represented a true breakthrough in the struggle to identify the causes of disease. Koch argued that to adequately attribute cause to an agent. the following criteria must be satisfied:

The agent must be identified in each case of the disease.

It must be produced in pure culture.

Introduction of the products of this culture into healthy animals must produce disease.

The agent must be cultured from the new host.

This was a far different level of proof than the convoluted theories that had formed debates on disease etiology for generations. Speculations about the origins of miasmas, the constitutional characteristics that predisposed to illness, the social prejudices that masqueraded as causal factors, the crude approximations of climate and geography that were thought to offer solutions to the conundrum of cause all wilted in the light of Koch's powerful experimental methods.

The inscrutable puzzle of consumption was beginning to yield. Koch's *bacillus*, as the new bacterium came to be known, begins its infective peregrinations in droplets from a cough, sneeze, or even conversation. Each drop contains 1 to several of the waxy, rod-shaped bacteria. Large numbers of these moist particles can be launched with every sneeze or utterance. Most of the droplets generated are too heavy for sustained flight and fall harmlessly to earth. Some smaller particles, however, dry out and float for hours. These are inhaled by the unwary, and the smallest particles make their way to the tiny alveoli, or air sacs of the lungs.

Once implanted there, the germs begin to slowly multiply, attracting in the process the attention of the host's immune cells. A battle ensues. Sometimes the immune system prevails and the invaders are destroyed. Occasionally, the bacteria gain a clear upper hand, multiplying and spreading to neighboring parts of the lung and other tissues in the body. More often, it is a standoff; the small nodules or tubercles are formed in which the bacteria hide, contained but still capable of mischief weeks, months, or even years later.

Tuberculosis has two distinct stages: infection and disease. Infection occurs when droplet nuclei are inhaled and set up habitation in the host. Because tuberculosis is acquired almost exclusively by the respiratory route, infection requires exposure to someone who is actively transmitting the bacteria. It turns out that though the disease is communicable, it is not highly so. Transmission is most likely when there is prolonged, close contact between individuals— most typically in households. Even then, infection may occur in 50% or fewer of household contacts. The extent of close contact and the quantity of organisms produced by the cough or sneeze are the 2 factors most related to the likelihood of infection.

Not everyone who is infected with the tuberculous bacillus comes down with disease. In fact, most do not. The cells of the immune system are successful in containing the germ about 90% of the time. Sometimes the invading organisms are completely eliminated, but more often, they are simply encircled and contained. This containment may last a lifetime. Only 10% of infected individuals are destined to come down with active tuberculosis. Chances of disease are greatest in the first few years following infection, though the risk persists for many years. Not infrequently a "new case" of tuberculosis in an older individual represents, not a recent exposure, but reactivation of a latent infection from the past.

In America, the report of Koch's discovery received a mixed reception. Among those committed to belief in the constitutional, hereditary nature of tuberculosis, the news was largely dismissed. One of Trudeau's teachers and mentors, Dr. Loomis, simply remarked that "he didn't much believe in germs" (4, p. 175). Trudeau, however, was exhilarated by the discovery. Having seen brief abstracts of the work in American journals, he was eager to read Koch's entire monograph. Unfortunately, Trudeau could not read German, and English versions were not available. He was rescued from frustration by a publisher friend from Philadelphia, who, hearing of his plight, organized the translation of Koch's work and presented it to the doctor in a large, handwritten copybook as a Christmas present. It was the start of Trudeau's pursuit of the cure for tuberculosis.

Convinced of the far-reaching importance of Koch's find, Trudeau was "intensely anxious" to replicate and extend the work. Undeterred by his total ignorance of bacteriology (the study of bacteria), he returned to New York City to learn all he could of the new discipline. This endeavor accomplished, he constructed a tiny, crude laboratory in a corner of his home and launched his efforts as a medical researcher (see Figure 6-3). He created artificial culture media from sheep's blood to propagate the tuberculosis bacillus and, soon, was able to isolate the bacteria from his patients to confirm that they had tuberculosis. But this work had all been done before. Trudeau had greater plans. His desire was to "inoculate animals and try experiments to destroy the germ" (4, p. 203).

His efforts were not successful. He injected guinea pigs and rabbits with his cultivated bacteria, then treated them with substances known to destroy the germs. Among these agents were creosote and Lister's carbolic acid. Unfortunately, as Trudeau reported, "the tubercle bacillus bore cheerfully a degree of medication which proved fatal to its host" (4, p. 204). Undaunted, he embarked on another question, one that had consumed him for some time. Ever since he had first come to the Adirondacks as a patient himself, Trudeau had pondered "how a change of climate, rest, fresh air, and food could influence the disease" (4, p. 205).

Fifteen rabbits were recruited to address the question. One group of 5 was inoculated with pure cultures of tuberculosis bacilli, then set loose on a small island to run wild in the fresh air and sunshine. A second group was similarly inoculated with tuberculosis

FIGURE 6-3

Dr. Trudeau in His Laboratory

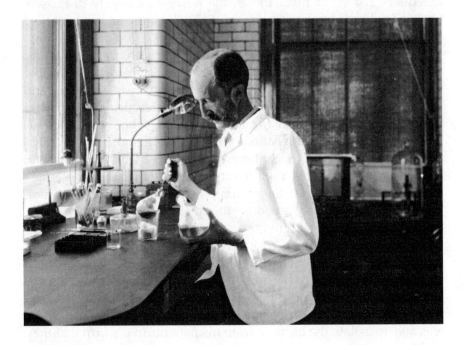

Source: Trudeau Institute Archives.

germs but confined in a dark, damp pit where the air was bad and food was insufficient. A third cohort of 5 was spared the tuberculosis inoculation but accommodated in the same unfavorable environment as group 2.

The results were reaffirming. Four of the 5 rabbits that enjoyed the sunshine, good food, and freedom survived despite their doses of bacillus. Group 2 had opposite results; 4 of the 5 subjected to the unfavorable surroundings died within 3 months. Examination of their organs after death revealed extensive tuberculosis. All group 3 rabbits survived and, though emaciated, were without tuberculous disease. Trudeau was delighted.

> This showed me conclusively that bad surroundings of themselves could not produce tuberculosis, and when once the germs had gained access to the body the course of the disease was greatly influenced by a favorable or unfavorable environment. The essence of sanitorium [sic] treatment

was a favorable environment so far as climate, fresh air, food, and regulation of the patient's habits were concerned, and I felt greatly encouraged as to the soundness of the method of treatment the Sanitarium represented, even though it did not aim directly at the destruction of the germ. (4, pp. 205–206)

Indeed, it was a fine experiment—well controlled, with a non-infected comparison group—reminiscent of Waterhouse and his experiment with vaccination. Of course, these were rabbits, not people, and as Trudeau readily admitted, sanitarium treatment "did not aim directly at the destruction of the germ" (4, pp. 205–206). His next attempts were even more ambitious:

> I began to realize about this time that the direct destruction of the germ in the tissues by germicides was a hopeless proposition and, inspired by Pasteur's work….I sought to produce immunity in my animals by dead germs, or preventive inoculations of substances derived from the liquid cultures from which the bacilli had been filtered. (4, p. 212)

He set to work immunizing guinea pigs and rabbits, hoping to actually prevent the disease.

Trudeau was not alone in this idea. Robert Koch had continued working on tuberculosis after he first isolated the bacteria. He, too, had been searching for remedies. In August 1890, just 3 months before Trudeau would publish his results on immunizing guinea pigs, Koch announced that he had created a substance that not only protected animals against tuberculosis but brought active disease to a complete standstill. Koch stopped short of claiming his discovery cured the disease in humans, but for a world desperate for relief, the extrapolated conclusions were predictable. Trudeau described the response at the Adirondack Cottage Sanitarium:

> It would be hard to exaggerate the intense excitement that pervaded the little colony of invalids at Saranac Lake when Koch's first announcement of his specific was published in the daily press, and I had all I could do to prevent several of my patients from rushing over to Berlin at once to be cured. (4, pp. 212-213)

Trudeau waited impatiently for details of the experiments, for the "recipe" of the successful cure or at least for samples of "Koch's lymph" so that he might treat his own patients. Koch, however, was slow to tell the world just how he made his lymph. Months lapsed until, under great pressure, he revealed the nature of his discovery. When finally Koch disclosed that the substance was nothing more than a glycerin extract of tuberculous bacillus, Trudeau was shocked. The material was almost identical to the substance he had used to immunize his guinea pigs. It became known as *tuberculin*. The difference was, Trudeau's experiments had shown no benefit.

It was a blow to Trudeau's faith in the deified Dr. Koch. Reports from others on tuberculin added to the concern. Patients injected with the substance frequently had strong reactions, including high fevers, and improvement did not follow.

Most physicians abandoned tuberculin soon after its frequent ill effects were appreciated. A few, Trudeau among them, continued to experiment with the "lymph" in hopes that Koch's promise would be fulfilled. By 1900, Trudeau was able to report on the results of almost 50 of his patients to whom he had administered tuberculin. All had been discharged as "cured" from the sanitarium. Forty-one of the 47 he could trace were well; only 6 had relapsed or were dead. That was an 87% rate of success.

The results seemed promising. But Trudeau recognized that the course of tuberculosis was variable and all his subjects had also experienced his sanitarium treatment. It was unclear how much additional benefit tuberculin conferred. So he compared results of his tuberculin-treated patients with 50 who were untreated but also discharged as apparently cured. And 77% of them remained well. Though the comparison showed "a slight percentage in favor of the tuberculin cases," Trudeau correctly recognized that the small difference was "not sufficiently marked to be in any way conclusive" (9).

It was a step in the right direction—the use of a control or comparison group. It was a strategy reminiscent of Waterhouse and the cowpox experiment of almost one hundred years before. Trudeau recognized that his comparison was not perfect. Ideally, the control should resemble experimental subjects in every feature save the receipt of treatment. But, as we have already seen with the sick or elderly who were given influenza vaccine and the healthier women who take hormone replacement therapy, people given treatment often differ from those who don't receive it in ways that relate to the outcome. Trudeau notes: "Some little allowance however, must be made for the fact that...that those treated with tuberculin were selected with special care" (9). When Trudeau evaluates the overall results, he finds that outcomes are heavily influenced by patient status on admission. As Table 6-1 indicates, his "incipient," or very mild, cases fare much better than far advanced cases –98% cured or improved versus 64%. If tuberculin administration is indeed supplied to those most likely to have favorable outcomes to begin with, favorable results are not surprising.

Controls provide a background rate of spontaneous recovery (or decline) and some estimate of the role of external influences on the course of illness. A landmark example of the importance of controls is a British Medical Research Council (MRC) study conducted in the 1940s to test a remedy for tuberculosis. The investigation was based on knowledge that a mold called streptomycin had killed a variety of bacteria in laboratory cultures. The new *antibiotic* showed promise as a drug to fight a number of infections in humans— among them, tuberculosis. The MRC investigators found over 100 tuberculosis subjects for their experiment. Patients were only included if they had "acute, progressive, bilateral pulmonary tuberculosis" for which the "estimated chances of spontaneous regression must be small" (10). All were placed on compete bed rest and close medical supervision. Fifty-five of the subjects were allocated to receive the active drug, streptomycin, and 52 had bed rest only. The results of the study are shown in Table 6-2.

The trial was a resounding success. Substantially more patients recovered and fewer died among those receiving the antibiotic than among controls. The experiment marked the beginning of our modern era of evidence-based medical therapeutics. However, the data

TABLE 6-1

Patients Who Remained an Average of 8-3/4 Months (Percent)

Condition of Patient When Admitted	Disease Cured/ Arrested/Improved	Unimproved or Failed	Died
113 incipient cases	98	2	0
151 advanced cases	91	9	1
59 far advanced cases	64	27	8
323 total			

Source: Based on Trudeau (9).

TABLE 6-2

Status of Tuberculosis 12 Months After Admission [Number (Percent)]

Group	Improvement	No Change	Deterioration	Death
Streptomycin (55)	31 (56)	4 (7)	8 (15)	12 (22)
Control (52)	16 (31)	5 (10)	7 (13)	24 (46)

Source: From British Medical Research Council (10).

also reaffirmed lessons on the variability of disease. Even though TB patients were selected because of the severity and progressive nature of their disease, 31% of those in the *untreated* group improved. At the same time, not all patients receiving the antibiotic were therapeutic successes: 15% showed deterioration in their disease and 22% died.

Another limitation to Trudeau's experiment is that all his study subjects are patients at the sanitarium. All are receiving the benefits of fresh air, rest, and improved nutrition. Trudeau would expect some improvement from these other sources. One can't assess the contribution of tuberculin when more than one potential therapy is being applied. Are patients improving because of tuberculin, because of the fresh air, or simply "on their own"? Trudeau believed passionately that the curative powers of his sanitarium were chiefly responsible. In truth, he actually had little sound evidence that his treatment actually cured the disease. His personal emergence from death's door and complete financial and emotional commitment to the Adirondack Cottage project scarcely makes him an unbiased evaluator.

The rise of the American sanatorium corresponded with a dramatic fall in tuberculosis mortality. In 1900 (the first year of reliable national data), 194 deaths from tuberculosis were recorded for every 100,000 people. By 1950, the rate had fallen to 22 per 100,000 people. It is tempting to link the trends in a causal fashion. But that would not be wise. Trends, as we have seen with Shattuck, may present an honest view of changing states of health, but assigning responsibility for the change is tricky. Often multiple elements are at play.

Increasing availability of sanatorium treatment in the years after the Adirondack Cottage opened may be an obvious change in tuberculosis care. But there were others. The general well being of the United States population was improving. Overall death rates were falling as well (although not as rapidly as TB rates). There were also improvements in housing, nutrition, and working conditions, each of which could be expected to assist the population's resistance to tuberculosis. Understanding of the contagious nature of the disease also increased. This meant that physicians began to diagnose cases earlier, observe family contacts more carefully, and reduce further contact by quarantine and isolation.

New technology also helped. Tuberculin, though failing as a remedy, proved a useful diagnostic aid. The inflammation provoked by small doses injected in the skin (a sign of the host's immune reactivity and reason for the serious reactions patients experienced with "treatment" doses) identified people who were infected but who might still be without clinical signs of disease. The x-ray tube discovered by Roentgen in 1895 gave doctors views inside the patient's chest, where shadows of incipient infection lurked.

Public health departments, first established after the Civil War following Shattuck's model, had taken on greater substance and authority and now promulgated regulations to decrease the spread of tuberculosis. Hermann Biggs, of the New York City Health Department, tackled tuberculosis with a vengeance. His model for comprehensive control included mandatory reporting of tuberculosis cases to the health department, follow-up of infected individuals by nurses, and extensive public education efforts. Regulations were enacted that made forced confinement of infectious patients possible and recognized the dangers of "promiscuous spitting" by forbidding it "upon the floors of buildings and of railroad cars and of ferry-boats" (11, pp. 141–142).

Even surgery contributed to the effort. For some years it had been observed that, among tuberculous individuals whose lungs had inadvertently collapsed from wounds that pierced the chest, the disease became arrested or improved. By the early 1900s, surgeons were deliberately collapsing lungs by injecting air into the pleural space just inside the chest wall.

All these changes are competing interventions that might contribute to the falling TB rates. When these occur concurrently, isolating any single one and designating it as responsible for vanquishing tuberculosis is impossible. *Cointerventions*, intentional or unintentional, recognized or unrecognized, are almost inevitable when observing health trends in human society. They represent another obstacle to identifying efficacy and are another reason why equivalent control groups are essential.

Another potent distraction from deciding on the efficacy of therapy is the natural, healthy desire of sick people to get well. The *placebo effect* is observed when there is an improvement in a subject's condition that is due, not to the treatment itself, but to the idea of or belief in treatment. "I shall please" is the literal translation of placebo from its Latin origins. The effect occurs, not because of the direct chemical or physiological activity of a particular drug or procedure, but because it is mediated through the treatment's psychological impact. The placebo effect is potent and can be quite helpful. When people are ill, any boost to their ability to improve is a good thing. Nevertheless, this boost is not useful when we are attempting to isolate the role of treatment in the course of disease.

One of the first people to document the extent of the placebo effect was a Boston researcher named Henry Beecher. In the mid-1950s Beecher cataloged 15 examples of medical studies where the effect was evident (12). He identified over 1000 subjects with conditions ranging from anxiety and tension to common colds, seasickness and headache to severe postoperative wound pain and chest pain due to heart disease. On average, he concluded, placebos provided relief from the problem about 35% of the time.

To reduce the confusion introduced by placebos one must not only include control subjects but have subjects who believe that they may have been treated. An inactive or sham therapy is given, the proverbial "sugar pill." We encountered placebo treatment in Chapter 3 when saltwater injections were administered to subjects who served as comparisons for cold vaccine recipients. Placebos are relatively easy to supply when treatments are packaged in the form of tablets or injections. The task becomes a bit more challenging, however, when complex treatments, such as a surgical procedure, are involved.

In one bold example, conducted in the 1950s, a group of investigators performed sham operations on subjects suffering from severe chest pain due to heart disease. The condition that prompted surgery, known as angina pectoris, afflicts thousands of men and women. Pain is brought on by exercise or exertion and is relieved by rest. It occurs when the heart receives an inadequate supply of blood to perform its pumping obligations. This situation arises because of narrowing of the coronary (heart) arteries from fatty deposits or plaques. The knowledge that the body sometimes produces new blood vessels when existing arteries become compromised prompted doctors to theorize that *deliberately* restricting the flow of several "nonessential" vessels near the heart might stimulate new growth that would enhance supply to the myocardium (that is, the heart muscle). A surgical procedure was developed in which internal mammary arteries that lie beneath the breastbone, near the heart, were surgically isolated and tied off to initiate this supplemental blood flow.

Results obtained from early experiments, conducted without controls, were inspiring. In one report of operations on 50 angina patients, two-thirds noted improvement. And 36% reported that their pain had ceased entirely following the operation (13). It was a remarkable result, almost too good to be true. Skeptical colleagues, aware of both the variability of angina attacks as well as the strong placebo effect associated with treatment as dramatic as surgery, agree. The benefits of the operation were "too good to be true."

The skeptics produced their own experiment, this time including control subjects (14). For each angina patient whose arteries were tied, another subject underwent preoperative preparation, local anesthesia, incisions through the chest wall, and isolation of the internal mammary artery. But these vessels were not tied. Subjects were stitched back together and returned to the recovery room as if they had experienced the same procedure as their colleagues. And for the most part, they had. They had missed only the critical artery ligation.

In the 6 months following surgery, both "ligated" and "sham operation" patients were evaluated for improvement. In addition to self-reports, exercise tests on a treadmill were performed to document increased performance. Results for the 17 patients included in the trial are shown in Table 6-3.

Over 50% of subjects reported a greater than 40% improvement in their angina symptoms—in both groups. Two subjects

TABLE 6-3

Characteristics and Outcomes of Angina Pectoris Patients
with Ligation and Nonligation of Internal Mammary Arteries

Subject Group	Average Age	Sex Male/Female	Average Exercise Tolerance (min.)*		Reported Improvement (no. Patients)†	
			Before Operation	After Operation	>40%	None
Ligated	64	3/5	2.0	2.3	5	3
Non-ligated	54	9/0	2.8	3.8	5	2

*Standardized treadmill test for 10 minutes, or onset of chest pain.
†Patient's estimate of improvement in angina afforded by operation.
Source: Based on Cobb (14).

improved on the treadmill to the point where they walked the entire 10 minutes allotted time without experiencing chest pain; both were in the "sham" group. The findings do not support the purported benefits of the operation. They do indicate the potency of the placebo effect. Even severe chest pain, associated with diagnosed heart disease, can be influenced by the power of the mind.

It should not need saying that subjects should be unaware of whether they are receiving active or placebo treatment. Such knowledge would defeat the entire purpose of a placebo control. Keeping subjects *blind* to their treatment status in an experiment is essential. They must not know whether they are receiving saltwater or the "real" cold vaccine. That is not always an easy task. In another experiment that attacked the problem of the common cold, a breakdown in blinding created problems in interpretation.

Investigators in this trial chose employees of the National Institutes of Health (NIH), our country's premiere research establishment, for their subjects (15). Some subjects were given capsules of ascorbic acid (vitamin C); others were provided with look-alike capsules containing lactose (milk sugar). Subjects were then observed to see how many colds they contracted in succeeding months and how long each cold lasted. Although the trial was properly designed to guard against the placebo effect, the study subjects were not entirely cooperative. NIH employees are by nature an inquisitive lot.

A number could not resist opening and tasting their capsules. Many correctly guessed, based on the sour taste of ascorbic acid, whether they were receiving the vitamin C or the placebo. The trial lost its blinding. When researchers analyzed the results, they found that, while the number of colds experienced by subjects in the two groups was similar, the typical duration of colds was significantly shorter among those receiving vitamin C. That could have been a promising result. However, when the problem of "unblinding" was taken into account and results were analyzed according to whether subjects had guessed the identity of their drug, only unblinded subjects displayed the diminution in duration of colds. For subjects who remained unaware of their treatment status, there was no difference.

There has been continuing controversy over the use of placebo treatments in human trials. Is it ethical to give ill subjects a compound that is without physiologic effect? Indeed, if an inactive treatment is given to individuals when one of known efficacy is available, it is an unethical situation. The critical requirement in an ethical experiment is that the treatment under evaluation is of *unknown* benefit. Clearly, investigators must have reason to believe the new treatment will work. These expectations may be based on animal experiments or limited, uncontrolled trials on humans. But the evidence at the time of the trial must be inconclusive. There must be uncertainty about the value of the new therapy. The expectation of benefit and uncertainty of efficacy justify the use of a placebo group. Without the placebo or sham, the influence of the strong desire among patients and investigators alike to see improvement creates bias and critically impairs our ability to judge treatment efficacy.

It's also important that the subjects who receive active treatment and those who are given placebo are as similar to one another as possible in every way except their treatment status. If subjects who are healthier to begin with or sicker from the start are more likely to become active treatment subjects than controls, results will be compromised.

We saw back in Chapter 3, in the natural experiment on flu vaccination, that the older patients in Minnesota were more likely to receive flu vaccine when they had chronic diseases. They were thus at greater risk for the outcome, hospitalization, than comparison subjects who did not receive vaccine. Efficacy of the flu vaccine was likely underestimated because of this selection bias. On the obverse side, women taking hormone replacement therapy were seen to be basically healthier than those not taking estrogens, so that potential benefits on heart disease might be attributable to factors other than the hormone replacement.

Ideally, active treatment and placebo control groups should be identical with respect to characteristics that place them at risk for the outcome of interest (such as hospitalization or heart disease). That can be a tall order. Some risk characteristics, such as age or other medical conditions, are obvious and may be clearly related to outcomes. But there may be others, such as healthier lifestyle or nuances in diet that are less readily identified and captured. Moreover, to catalog all the potential characteristics of subjects that might relate to outcome and apportion these evenly between treatment and control groups is an almost impossible task.

There is a solution. It's known as *random allocation*. With random allocation, every subject in an experiment has an equal chance of being placed in the active treatment or the control group. Assignment is determined by chance—a "flip of the coin" or, more properly, using a table of random numbers. The idea is to avoid potential bias either by investigators assigning patients or by patients preferentially choosing their group. Prior to study entry, subjects must agree to this random allocation scheme. Once assigned, they and investigators must remain unaware of the assignment until the experiment is concluded. When this all happens according to plan, we have a *randomized, double-blind trial*.

Random allocation removes bias from patient assignment. Unfortunately, it doesn't guarantee that similarity in treatment and control populations will be achieved. While we can have confidence that subject's selective willingness and investigators' hopes for a "good result" are discouraged by random allocation, it is a procedure that depends upon chance. And as anyone who has flipped a coin will attest, an equal number of heads and tails in a trial of 10 tosses doesn't always occur. We may get 6 heads and 4 tails or 7 tails and 3 heads. The proportions can vary substantially with such a small number of tosses. So it is with subject allocation. In experiments with relatively small numbers of subjects, characteristics of the groups may not balance when chance alone is operating.

Consider the mammary artery ligation trial. The number of subjects in this experiment was small—only 17. And, even though there was proper random allocation, the active and sham groups were not comparable (review Table 6-3). Average age differed between the groups, as did the proportion of males to females. Because these factors are known to be related to the outcome (less chest pain), interpretation of the results is clouded. Though the results indicated no apparent improvement in chest pain following the surgery, a question remains whether differences in the baseline risks of the two subject groups might have obscured a benefit.

Random allocation can never guarantee comparability among study subject groups. However, one is more likely to see patient characteristics equilibrate when the number of subjects in a study is large. If a trial of coin tosses includes 100 flips, it is more probable that a result approaching the anticipated 50% heads and 50% tails will be achieved. Experimental studies always run the risk of unbalanced allocation, even when bias has been controlled. Knowledgeable researchers, understanding this problem, will routinely evaluate the distribution of important patient risk-subject risk characteristics following random allocation to see if subject risks are balanced between the experimental and comparison groups.

The well-conducted British MRC trials of streptomycin clarified longstanding puzzles relating to tuberculosis treatment. Other studies soon followed and more effective antibiotics became available. At the same time, new observational studies were adding complexity to our understanding of the cause of tuberculosis. With the surge of the "microbiologic revolution" in the latter 19th and early 20th centuries came the conviction that understanding causes of disease was an easy matter. One had only to follow Koch's guidelines to identify and culture a responsible microorganism. A germ lurked behind every disease and only waited to be discovered.

It turned out things were not so simple. By the middle of the 20th century, researchers were engaged in questions of why tuberculosis had such a variable course in different individuals—why some infected people get sick and others ward off the disease. Ironically, their findings returned full circle to the notions of

100 years before: Genetics and environmental factors, both physical and social, turned out to be important after all. While many harbored tuberculous bacilli in their bodies, the germ turns out to be a *necessary* but not sufficient determinant of disease.

Overcrowded living conditions and poor nutrition were confirmed as risks that lead to disease. That finding makes sense. Overcrowding creates increased exposure to the transmissible bacteria. Poor nutrition decreases the body's resistance. But other factors in the social environment were also shown to play a role.

In the 1950s, a group of investigators from the University of Washington addressed the centuries-old belief that tuberculosis was initiated by unhappy or stressful life experiences (16). Recognizing that conducting an experiment in which subjects were deliberately subjected to stress was out of the question, they applied their best efforts to approximate an experimental design using an observational or "real-life" setting.

They found a suitable group of subjects among the employees at Firland Sanatorium, a TB treatment facility located in Washington State. It was a clever choice. Employees at the sanatorium were all exposed to tuberculosis. Because of that exposure, they were closely observed (including periodic examinations and chest radiographs) throughout the course of their employment.

Among the group, 20 individuals were identified who had developed active pulmonary tuberculosis. For comparison, the researchers found 20 other employees who were similar to the cases. They were of the same sex, race, job classification, employment duration, and decade of age as tuberculosis subjects. This is *matching*—selecting comparison subjects so that specific characteristics are similar to cases. Matching reduces or *controls* these factors as potential explanations of illness, since the factors are similar in both groups.

A questionnaire was given to each group. The items probed for the occurrence of stressful life events. Included were such difficulties as financial hardship, change of job, residence relocation, change in social relationships, and work or marital stress. Questions related to a subject's experience over a 10-year period, but the investigators were most interested in events that occurred within the 2 years just prior to the onset of tuberculous disease. Both groups reported stressful occurrences. Over the entire 10 years, the control group actually identified a somewhat larger number than tuberculosis cases. But in the 2 years leading up to onset of disease, tuberculosis cases reported far more problems. Table 6-4 shows the comparison between the groups.

The authors conclude that "the employees who became ill did so in a situation of stress which would be conducive to lower resistance." The "cause" was not so simple after all. The presence of the TB bacillus was necessary for contracting the disease, but it was not the whole story, not sufficient by itself. Other factors in the patient's social, physical, and emotional environment play a critical role in the development of the disease, as the Firland experience shows. The causes of human disease are seldom single or simple. Most often there are multiple, linked components—chains or webs that create cause.

The TB story is remarkably instructive. For many years, the etiology of the disease was subject to the same disputes—miasma versus contagion, environment versus moral character—that accompanied the illnesses we have examined previously. The hereditary

TABLE 6-4

Proportion of the Frequency of Each Item Group of the Schedule of Recent Experience Appearing in the Final 2 Years for 20 Tuberculous and 20 Matched Nontuberculous Employees of Firland Sanatorium

Item Group	Mean Percentage Recorded in the Final 2 Years	
	Tuberculous	Nontuberculous
Financial hardship	29.8	8.1
Job changes	30.1	6.2
Residence changes	31.7	4.9
Changes in social relations	35.5	22.7
Irregular habits	28.8	9.4
Personal crisis	68.1	20.0
Work stress	33.3	11.3
Marital stress	40.0	33.3

Source: Based on Hawkins (16).

hypothesis that emerged was favored by medical and nonmedical minds alike. As with the other theories, it had a basis in human experience.

The principal evidence, provided by the stories of the Shattucks and the Emersons, was the repeated observation that high rates of consumption "ran" in families. Clustering of illness among the crowded, slum-dwelling poor reinforced the idea of constitutional predisposition (and was consistent with other prejudices against the under-privileged as possessing character defects as well). The observations supporting the link between heredity and tuberculosis were accurate. It did occur in families, and rates were higher among the urban poor. What was not considered, however, were alternative explanations for these findings. Family members live in close contact. So do the poor. The link was not inborn susceptibility but proximity itself. The longer and closer the contact between a person with a contagious disease and a susceptible individual, the more likely is transmission. It is a principle that seems obvious to us now, but it eluded most Victorian minds. Family membership and poverty are simply markers of a common causal element—close contact. They are not causes of tuberculosis.

From America's greatest 19th-century killer, tuberculosis has fallen to a minor cause of mortality. When Trudeau was born, a century and a half ago, tuberculosis was responsible for almost 1 death in every 4; it now accounts for less than 1 in every 2400. Now, fewer than 6 new cases of the disease occur each year per 100,000 population, the lowest rate since incidence (new cases per unit of population per year) has been recorded. Globally, however, the disease still haunts us. Over 8 million new cases and 2 million deaths occur each year. Sub-Saharan Africa and Southeast Asia are most afflicted, and the trends are not encouraging.

In 1915, Edward Trudeau succumbed to the disease he had battled with such personal and professional passion for so long. The American sanatorium movement he had founded flourished over the ensuing 30 years, only to be rendered obsolete by the miracle of antibiotics. In the first years of the 20th century, when Trudeau's work was gathering a national following, facilities dedicated to the treatment of tuberculosis were sparse. In 1900, there were 34 facilities, capable of caring for fewer than 4500 patients, across the country. During the next 50 years, the numbers swelled to over 800 hospitals and sanatoria, both public and private, with over 130,000 beds assigned to tuberculosis (5, p. 198). As antibiotic treatment took over, the facilities closed entirely or were converted to other uses-long-term care or treatment of other chest diseases. The Trudeau Sanatorium discharged its last patient in 1954.

Trudeau's ultimate contribution to the control of tuberculosis was probably more spiritual than scientific. His research yielded few new insights and his therapeutic recipe of fresh air, rest, and proper diet may or may not have been effective. Yet his personal struggle with tuberculosis, his endless energy, and his dedication inspired many. He was an elegant spokesperson at a dramatic turning in our thinking about disease. "This time in medicine," he wrote toward the end of his life, "was the dawn of the achievements of the new experimental method—a method which was casting so much light on dark places—and the glamour of its possibilities in the prevention and cure of disease took a strong hold on my imagination" (4, p. 174). Trudeau presided at the greatest paradigm shift in public health. In his "hour," consumption, the enigmatic, romanticized affliction that cast its shadow of despair across the 19th century was transformed. It became comprehensible. It was still deadly but could be understood. Tuberculosis was an infection, brought on by microscopic particles which could be stained and grown in laboratories by medical scientists who, as things were going, might one day master it.

REFERENCES

1. Shattuck L. *Lemuel Shattuck Papers*, 1805–1867, Massachusetts Historical Society, Boston.
2. Shattuck L. *Report of the Sanitary Commission of Massachusetts 1850*. Cambridge: Harvard University Press; 1948.
3. Alcott LM. *Little Women*. New York: Modern Library; 1983.
4. Trudeau EL. *An Autobiography*. Garden City, New York: Doubleday Page & Company; 1915.

5. Rothman SA. *Living in the Shadow of Death*. New York: Basic Books; 1994.

6. Drake D, Levine ND. *Malaria in the Interior Valley of North America*. Urbana: University of Illinois Press; 1964.

7. Lister J. On the antiseptic principle of the practice of surgery. *Lancet*. 1867; 2:353–356.

8. Dubos R, Dubos J. *The White Plague*. Boston: Little, Brown & Company; 1952.

9. Trudeau EL. The sanitarium treatment of incipient pulmonary tuberculosis, and its results. *Transactions of the Association of American Physicians*. 1900; 15:36–47.

10. British Medical Research Council. Streptomycin treatment of pulmonary tuberculosis, a Medical Research Council investigation. *Brit Med J*. 1948:769–772.

11. Winslow CEA. *The Life of Hermann M. Biggs, Physician and Statesman of the Public Health*. Philadelphia: Lea & Febiger; 1929.

12. Beecher HK. The powerful placebo. *J Am Med Assoc*. Dec. 24 1955; 159:1602–1606.

13. Kitchell R, Glover RP, Kyle RH. Bilateral internal mammary artery ligation for angina pectoris. *Amer J Cardiol*.1958:46–50.

14. Cobb LA, Thomas GI, Dillard DH, Merendino AK, Bruce RA. An evaluation of internal-mammary-artery ligation by a double-blind technic. *N Engl J Med*. 1959; 260:1115–1118.

15. Karlowski TR, Chalmers TC, Frenkel LD, Kapikian AZ, Lewis TL, Lynch JM. Ascorbic acid for the common cold. *JAMA*. 1975; 231:1038–1042.

16. Hawkins N, Davies R, Holmes T. Evidence of psychosocial factors in the development of pulmonary tuberculosis. *Amer Rev Tuberculosis*. 1957; 75:768–779.

CHAPTER 7

The Beginning
and the End:
Epidemic Poliomyelitis

In the summer of 1894, the microbiologic revolution was fully in flower. Twelve years had passed since Koch had announced that the rod-shaped bacillus that now bore his name was the cause of tuberculosis. The list of diseases that could now be linked to particular, provoking microorganisms was growing rapidly. In addition to anthrax and tuberculosis, Koch had added the germ that caused the epidemic, diarrheal disease, cholera. Laveran, as we noted in Chapter 4, contributed the parasite responsible for malaria in 1880. The contaminated wounds that Lister had prevented were found to be due to tiny grapelike clusters of a bacterium that was designated *staphylococcus*. Microbes responsible for leprosy, gonorrhea, relapsing fever, typhoid, and diphtheria were also on the list.

The field of immunology was budding, too. The tantalizing promise, first offered by smallpox vaccination, of preventing disease by artificially inducing immunity, was being fulfilled. In July 1885, a 9-year-old boy, who had been severely bitten by a rabid dog, was saved from certain death by immunizing injections given him by Pasteur. At the same time, a Russian zoologist named Elie Metchnikoff had discovered amoeboid cells within the blood that engulfed and rendered harmless foreign particles such as bacteria. Cell-free serum was also found to have antibacterial properties. Survivors of infection produced circulating substances that neutralized repeat invasions of a similar type. The excruciating muscle contractions of tetanus and

155

suffocating respiratory symptoms of diphtheria were discovered to be due to toxins produced by bacteria. When these toxins were injected into animals, antitoxins were produced—proteins that bound with the toxins to neutralize their ill effects. Treatments based on immunology were now in hand.

Few of these exciting medical triumphs concerned the residents of Vermont's Otter Creek region that summer. This tranquil New England valley, bounded by the Green Mountains on the east and the marble-laden Taconics to the west, sheltered 26,000 inhabitants from the larger world—its miracles and its maladies. They were farmers, quarrymen, and mill workers, from towns like Rutland and Procter. They were people who relished their distance from the populous, polluted coastal cities and rejoiced in their clean air, pure water, and robust health. So when the epidemic struck and the residents themselves became medical news, it was a cruel surprise. From mid-June until the first week in October 1894, 132 of them became statistics in the largest outbreak of its kind that had ever been reported—not just in Vermont but in the world. It was a new and terrifying illness. Neither cause nor means of spread were known, and 1 in every 7 of its victims died. Two features of the illness were particularly distressing: Its victims were primarily children and, though most recovered, many survivors were damaged—permanently disabled with weakened, withered arms and legs. The case of Patrick N. summary was typical:

> Boy, 3½ years, Irish. Hygienic surroundings fair; sturdy child; most active of a family of three children. Only apparent cause playing too hard on a hot day. Taken with high fever, temperature 102° F., nausea, general restlessness and headache....On third day acute symptoms subsided except the incontinence of urine. It was then noticed that he had lost the use of his legs. Patellar reflexes diminished and considerable hyperesthesia of the legs....The left leg improved rapidly, the right slowly. After six weeks was able to stand and take a few steps by taking hold of chairs. After three months the paralysis and wasting were confined to the right glutei [buttock] and lower spinal muscles. His efforts to walk have brought on a slight spinal curvature....The paralysis, however, persists in the glutei and lower spinal muscles and promises to be permanent. (1, pp 24–25)

In truth, this was not the first appearance of the disease. More than 100 years earlier, an English physician named Michael

Underwood had elegantly described the illness. There had also been reports in the American medical literature, but these were sporadic—seldom more than several at a time and almost always involving infants in the first few years of life. Then in the 1880s, several outbreaks of the paralytic disease were reported from Europe, Scandinavia in particular. The largest and best documented occurred in Sweden in 1887 and consisted of 44 cases.

The Otter Creek Valley outbreak was not only the largest that had been described, it was probably the best documented. The careful records of the cases were the work of a single, tireless individual, a Rutland physician named Charles Caverly (see Figure 7-1). A modest, mustached man, Caverly had a practice in Rutland, but he was also head of Vermont's State Board of Health. It was this responsibility and his sense of the "general feeling of uneasiness that was perceptible among the people in regard to the 'new disease' that was affecting the children," that he decided a systematic investigation was required (1; p. 15). Painstakingly, he gathered reports of all the cases in the

FIGURE 7-1

Charles Caverly

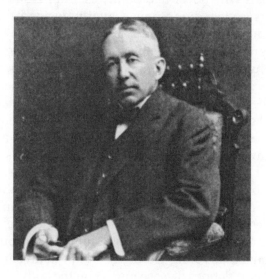

Source: Vermont Department of Public Health.

region, 132 in all. He then cast the data he extracted into tables describing the "when, where, who" of the epidemic.

The first case was noted on June 17 and the peak occurred August 1. It was a summer disease. Although the illness prevailed along the pathway of the Otter Creek, Caverly could find no relationship between the water supply and occurrence nor correlations with sanitary surroundings or socioeconomic status of victims. No geologic features of the valley informed his search for explanations. But the characteristics of the victims were more revealing. Ninety of the cases were less than 6 years of age; 15 were between the ages of 6 and 14; and 15 more were over 14 years of age. Nervous system and muscular complaints were common. Rigidity of the neck and back, headaches and sore muscles, hypersensitivity to touch, and general convulsions were all reported. The most striking feature was paralysis: It occurred in 119 of the cases. Legs and arms were most affected, sometimes singly, sometimes in combination. Paralysis of muscles of the tongue and face were also noted. There were 18 deaths. Caverly continued to track the cases in the months that followed; he found that 56 made complete recoveries. At least 30, however, had continuing paralysis 6 to 9 months later. One curious subgroup in his collection was made up of 6 individuals who never had paralysis. But because they all had other nervous system symptoms, Caverly decided they belonged to the epidemic. These became known as "abortive" cases. Later they would prove a crucial insight.

Local physicians were baffled by the illness, both its nature and its cause. Meningitis and neuritis were mentioned frequently, but not all the pieces fit. Caverly was better read than most doctors and well connected. He knew of the Scandinavian epidemics and had corresponded with America's best-known expert on the condition. Caverly concluded that the epidemic was due to *poliomyelitis*, more commonly known as *infantile paralysis*.

The double designation of the illness was significant, emblematic of the progress medical science was making. Infantile paralysis is a clinical description. The term simply identifies the major visible manifestation of the disease (paralysis) and the age group most often affected (infants and young children). But poliomyelitis is a pathologic diagnosis; it defines disease impact on the body's cells. Derived from *polios*, meaning gray, and *myelitis*, indicating inflammation of the spinal cord, the term describes the destruction of nerve cells that conduct impulses from the brain to the muscles. Beneath the microscope, these cells appear as "gray matter"; hence, the *polios*. With the loss of these cells, muscles are unable to contract or limbs to move. From the middle of the 1900s, there were great advances in identifying and describing the body's cellular structure in both normal and abnormal states and in correlating these with outward manifestations of disease. Microscopic anatomy and illness were being increasingly connected.

Several features of the illness were perplexing. Prior descriptions were almost entirely confined to infants and young children. Typically, 94% of cases were in children less than 6 years old, with only 1% above the age of 10. In fact, because he found so much illness among older children and adults, Caverly wondered whether the diagnosis was correct. Could one have "infantile paralysis" when the victims were not infants?

Other findings also puzzled him. The illness was rarely seen in more than one member of a family. Nor was Caverly able to link disease to the usual circumstances of poverty and poor sanitation. A likely causal candidate was a new bacterium or parasite, but shouldn't that mean spread in families and crowded neighborhoods? Why an epidemic in pristine Vermont? The facts didn't hang together.

Several of these features (older ages, few family clusters, and rural settings) had been seen before. A note in the Boston Medical and Surgical Journal of 1893 mentioned an apparent increase in the number of cases (26) of polio in the Boston area that summer. It reported that cases were dispersed throughout the suburbs but that very few came from Boston proper. The unusual age distribution had also been observed in Scandinavia. There, over half the cases were found to be above the age of 6 and numbers of adults were stricken (2, pp. 79–84).

It was 1910 when Caverly next wrote about poliomyelitis. Vermont had not suffered from the disease "in anything approaching epidemic form" in the interval since 1894. This was not the situation elsewhere:

> From 1894 to the present time this disease has increased with alarming rapidity—not only in this country but abroad. Many large epidemics have occurred and the death rate has apparently increased with the epidemic prevalence of the disease.

As would be expected of a disease that is so obviously spreading and recurring in epidemic form, poliomyelitis is being studied now the world over. (1, p. 39)

Indeed as the disease expanded, so did information about its cause and means of spread. In 1908, a Viennese immunologist named Karl Landsteiner induced poliomyelitis in monkeys by injecting them with bacteria-free material from the spinal cord of a fatal human case. The implications were both clear and profound. Poliomyelitis was transmissible, but its cause was not bacterial. A virus—not yet visible to even the most powerful microscope nor capable of being grown in laboratory culture—was responsible. Indirect identification was now possible; one could transfer polio in a laboratory animal. The following year (1909) Simon Flexner, of the Rockefeller Institute for Medical Research, replicated the experiment in New York. Flexner took the proof a step further by passing the disease from one monkey to another. The infectious, viral nature of polio seemed confirmed.

But the questions that perplexed Caverly remained. Despite the impressive laboratory evidence, the means by which polio spread through communities was still uncertain. It was one thing to transfer the virus by injecting monkeys with infected tissue, but quite another to explain polio's behavior in "the real world." The data were confusing and suggested that if polio were, indeed, contagious, it was not highly so. How else could one account the failure to connect outbreaks with crowded environments and poor sanitation, or with the infrequent occurrence of multiple cases within families? And what accounted for the shift in affected age groups?

The epidemic in Vermont in 1910 was only half the size of that of 1894, but Caverly's investigation was even more extensive. He collected data on nationality, on age of housing, on the soil condition about the house. He checked on the proximity to ponds, railways, and animal quarters, water supply, sewer facilities, and on the prior health of cases and their family members. He looked for cases that had recently been chilled, exposed to heat, immersed in water, or suffered recent injury. He tried his best to link the cases. None of these efforts proved fruitful. By now, however, Caverly was leaning toward accepting the role of contagion. "The disease is infectious, and, to a certain extent, contagious," he admitted, "it can probably be transmitted by third persons…as well as the sick." Then he noted, "inasmuch as there are various grades of severity of the disease, which we recognize by the paralysis, there are undoubtedly mild abortive cases" (1, pp. 53–54).

The concept of "abortive" cases intrigued him. Was it possible that people who were not sick could spread disease?

It took some years before there was agreement on the nature of transmission. Some remained convinced that polio was not contagious but due to an environmental toxin. Others, following the proof of mosquito propagation of malaria and yellow fever, believed that insect vectors held the key; flies were particularly suspect. Some, though favoring person-to-person communication, believed it was, like smallpox and tuberculosis, spread by the respiratory route. Ultimately, all these theories missed the mark.

Polio plays by different rules. It is, as we have come to understand, indeed initiated by a virus. But neither buzzing pests nor coughs nor sneezes are responsible for its spread. Polio infection comes through ingestion. The virus is swallowed. It first invades the tissues of the throat and tonsils, then the stomach and intestines. Once in residence, it migrates to lymph glands where it multiples, and eventually it can find its way into cells of the nervous system and spinal cord. From lodgings in the intestinal tract large amounts of virus are excreted in the feces; and it is fecal contamination that spreads the disease. This pattern of transmission is, like several other well-known epidemic diseases, such a cholera and typhoid, classed as "fecal-oral" spread. Lack of cleanliness and faulty sanitation are important factors in dissemination.

The first two decades of the 20th century saw increasing numbers of polio epidemics. In 1910, in addition to Vermont's second outbreak, there were epidemics in the rural Middle West. New York City was struck in 1907 and again in 1916. As experience with the disease increased, the inconsistent puzzle pieces began to join to create a plausible story. Caverly's attention to "abortive" cases proved critical. These suggested the disease presented as a spectrum of severity. If some infections resulted in only mild or inapparent illness, polio might be more prevalent in a community than was evident from the paralytic counts. This turned out to be the key.

We now appreciate that the great majority of people who are infected with polio virus do *not* become paralyzed. In fact, most don't even get sick; 95% of polio infections are inapparent or asymptomatic. Another 4% of those infected show only minor symptoms (sore throat and fever, nausea, and vomiting), symptoms indistinguishable from those of other less consequential "summer viruses." Less than 1% of polio virus infections result in paralysis of the arms and legs, or, most dramatically, the muscles controlling respiration. Even then, many who experience the loss of muscle function recover completely. The numbers who suffer the tragic, permanent crippling consequences of poliomyelitis represent a small fraction of those who are infected. For most, the immune system prevails, not only warding off adversity at the time but also providing safety from the illness in the future.

This *spectrum of disease* explains polio's confusing epidemic habits. The predilection of the early epidemics to rural, less populated areas rather than the urban slums now makes sense. Sanitation and hygiene *were* involved in the spread of polio—intimately in fact—but not in a pattern that had been seen before. Slums were ideal for spreading the virus. It was everywhere in these environments. That meant that almost everyone was exposed in infancy. By the time an individual reached the age of 6, infection and subsequent immunity were virtually assured. Sporadic or, endemic cases were routine. But as the paralytic complications of infections were infrequent (1%) and took place at an age where death and disability were already high, the problem was "invisible."

Where sanitation had improved and crowding was not universal, childhood spread was not the rule; some escaped early infection. These children remained susceptible and, as their number grew, so did the opportunity for epidemics. When virus is introduced into a community where the number of susceptibles (nonimmune individuals) is large, outbreaks erupt. Caverly's consternation that communicability and infrequency in families were incompatible can now be understood. Family members *were* affected. Most had inapparent or "aborted" infections.

The work of early health officers, like Charles Caverly, was seminal. Their carefully gathered data provided the critical clues to understanding poliomyelitis and became the model for epidemiologists who followed. Key to their approach was the thorough search for cases. Complete ascertainment was essential, not simply for the accuracy of numbers but for the need to uncover the disease in all its guises. Every illness presents a spectrum of manifestations and degrees of severity. In different individuals, the same virus or bacterium might produce a mild sore throat and low-grade fever or an upset stomach and a skin rash. It may result in just a few days of indisposition, or it might become a life-threatening crisis. If an exhaustive search for cases is not conducted, the range of illness might not be captured and a comprehensive picture of the disease not obtained. Had Caverly not been thorough, and insightful, he would have missed the mild, abortive cases that proved so central to unraveling the riddle of transmission.

The first few decades of the 20th century saw the viral cause of poliomyelitis confirmed and its person-to-person spread documented. Appreciation that provoking the immune system with weakened or inactivated agents could create protection from infection was also growing. Some immunologic method to protect from polio became an obvious priority. Efforts in this direction began as early as 1916. At first, the focus was on keeping those already ill from developing paralysis. *Serum therapy* was the first attempt. The approach was based upon the premise that the blood of recovered polio patients contained antibodies against the virus. When injected into polio patients in early stages of disease, these would neutralize the virus and ward off paralysis. The approach, now known as *passive immunization*, has been tried in many forms over the years. Techniques have varied from injecting human serum directly into the spinal canal, to intravenous infusions of antibody-rich horse serum, to jabbing 2 ounces of a parent's blood into a young child's buttock. Its most sophisticated form was gamma globulin, an antibody-rich fraction of human serum, that was widely used until the early 1950s.

Passive immunization was not successful. Some of the reasons are biological. Antibodies, which are programmed proteins directed against specific antigen invaders, have a limited life span. Their potency is lost in a matter of weeks. Given such a short life span, the logistics of timely administration become difficult. There is only a brief moment of opportunity, shortly before exposure to the virus or very soon after infection occurs, when gamma globulin can be expected to confer protection. Providing passive immunity to sufficient numbers of individuals in time to thwart an epidemic, or to household contacts early enough in their infection to ward off complications, proved too challenging.

Active immunization, stimulating the body to make its own protective antibodies, as Jenner had done with cowpox and Pasteur with rabies, offers a much better solution. Active immunity can be induced well in advance of impending exposure to an infectious agent and can be expected to protect for some years into the future. Several paths to active immunity are possible. One can try to weaken or *attenuate* the virus. Pasteur had created a less potent virus when he transferred rabies-infected brain tissue from animal to animal repeated times. The resulting virus was still capable of infecting cells, multiplying, and stimulating antibodies, but it had lost its *virulence*, the capacity to cause severe disease. Or, one could *inactivate* or kill the virus, rendering it incapable of multiplying but preserving enough of its recognizable antigenic structure to trigger antibody production in the host.

Problems are inherent in each approach. It is obviously imperative that any live attenuated vaccine is sufficiently weakened and, similarly, that a killed vaccine is truly inactive. The specter of injecting children with a virulent virus that causes rather than prevents an attack of polio is too distressing. Yet there was evidence that this had occurred. Two experiments conducted in the mid-1930s, one using an attenuated and one an inactivated virus, had produced at least a dozen cases of paralytic polio and 6 deaths (2). These experiments were widely criticized as overhasty, poorly executed efforts, and in their aftermath, the vaccine effort was untracked for over 2 decades.

There are also technical problems with producing virus for vaccines. For many years, the spinal cord and brain of monkeys was the only means of cultivating polio virus. Monkeys were expensive, difficult to handle, and, not infrequently, in short supply. It was, therefore, a breakthrough of some magnitude when, in 1948, Drs. John F. Enders, Thomas H. Weller, and Frederick S. Robbins from Boston found that polio virus could be grown in tissues other than the monkey's central nervous system. Skin and muscle cells from human embryos, which could be grown and maintained in laboratory cultures, supported its growth.

The path was now open for one of public health's landmark endeavors, the creation and evaluation of Jonas Salk's polio vaccine. Salk's work with polio began in 1948, when he took on responsibility for a large laboratory in Pittsburgh that was dedicated to identifying polio virus specimens.* Through this work, Salk's familiarity with the virus expanded and his techniques for propagating large amounts of polio in tissue cultures were perfected. Creation of a vaccine was only a matter of persistence. Salk was not an innovator. He was, however, a meticulous master of the laboratory. The haste that characterized the ill-fated 1935 vaccine experiments was not in his nature. He was a tireless perfectionist. No vaccine would leave his laboratory before its time. By 1953, Salk had tested a vaccine made from formalin-killed virus (the same chemical Lister had used to kill staphylococci) on several hundred human subjects with good results. Blood samples taken after immunization showed antibodies had been formed and no adverse effects had been reported.

It was none too soon. The world (both scientists and laymen) was desperate for relief from polio. The previous summer the disease produced unparalleled havoc; a record 22,000 paralytic cases were reported in the United States. The public was in panic. Swimming pools and summer camps and beaches closed. Amusement parks and movie theaters and even drinking fountains were declared "off limits." Almost any public contact was considered rife with risk. Specters of rows of massive, coffinlike respirators known as "iron lungs" (see Figure 7-2), each encasing a diminished human form that clung desperately to life, haunted every parent.

Most of Salk's colleagues were eager to proceed to larger trials to test the vaccine's effect. A few, like Dr. Albert Sabin, were less enthusiastic. Sabin thought that killed virus vaccine had little value; he favored waiting till an agent based on a live, attenuated strain could be produced. His reservations had some merit. Though Salk had shown that his vaccine could create antibodies, no one knew how long protection from a killed virus might last. But it was also true that Sabin's opposition was tinted by self-interest. Eight years Salk's senior, Sabin too dreamed of being the man to liberate the

---

* Polio virus was by this time known to exist as 3 antigenically distinct types with a number of different strains. This meant that any vaccine must stimulate antibodies against all 3 types to be successful.

FIGURE 7-2

Polio Patients in "Iron Lung" Respirators

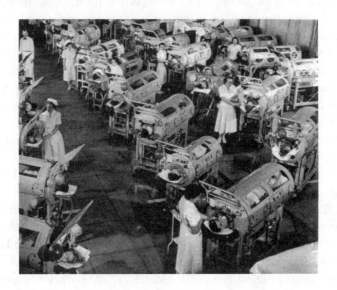

Source: March of Dimes Foundation.

world from poliomyelitis. Sabin had been a polio researcher much longer than Salk and he was working on attenuating the virus. Sabin frequently suggested that it was too early to embrace a plan for extensive trials of any killed vaccine, that at least 10 to 15 years more study would be required before such a vaccine would be ready. Sabin treated the "new man" with certain condescension, and rivalry between the two men grew as the race to test a vaccine intensified. Their differences had caused sparks at more than one scientific meeting.

What all could agree upon, however, was that, with the light of worldwide interest glaring on the project, the challenge became a dual one. Developing a vaccine that induced antibodies was only part of the effort. Planning and producing an adequate trial to test it in people was a second, perhaps more daunting, obstacle.

Previous efforts to evaluate polio preventatives had been marred by poor experimental design. Failures to guard against bias in subject selection and evaluation were common, and adequate use of comparison subjects was rare. It was imperative that the trial of Salk's vaccine not fall prey to such inadequacies. It was evident, however, that maintaining objectivity would be difficult. Pressure from the public and the press, as well as from the trial's sponsoring agency, the National Foundation for Infantile Paralysis, was intense. Everyone expected success and wanted it soon.

The man selected to lead the evaluation turned out to be the perfect choice. Dr. Thomas Francis was an accomplished virologist and epidemiologist. Widely respected for his work with the influenza virus, Francis was known to have unimpeachable scientific standards. He had been one of Jonas Salk's mentors. At the time Francis was approached to take on the evaluation of the trial, he was Director of the School of Public Health at the University of Michigan. He made it clear that, if he took the job, he would tolerate no interference in the evaluation—not from Jonas Salk, not from the National Foundation's dedicated but overbearing president, Basil O'Connor. A second, nonnegotiable demand was that the trial have a double-blind, placebo-controlled design. Once all parties agreed to the demand, the Salk vaccine evaluation became the francis tield trial.

The trial was an experiment of unprecedented scale in both planning and execution. Over 1.8 million children from 44 different states participated. Enlisted were 15,000 schools, and more than 150,000 individuals—doctors, nurses, physical therapists, teachers, health officers, virologists, epidemiologists and local volunteers—assisted the effort.

There were reasons why so many subjects were required and subtleties to designing the trial that are not immediately obvious. This was a *prevention* trial, not a *treatment* trial—an important distinction. In the British Medical Research Council treatment trial of streptomycin, (reported in Chapter 6) results were achieved with only 120 subjects. But these subjects already had tuberculosis, and the test was whether they improved after receiving the antibiotic. When children in the Francis field trial lined up to get their polio shots in the spring of 1954, no one was sick. The threat of illness still lay several months into the future. Nor was it certain that any of them would even be exposed to polio. There might or might not be epidemics in the communities in which the trial was taking place. Moreover, because so many polio infections are inapparent, it was likely that many of the children had already been exposed to polio and developed protective antibodies without the aid of vaccine. Francis estimated that only 10 to 20% of children in the targeted 6- to 9-year-old age group would be susceptible to the disease. It all meant that much larger numbers of subjects were required than would have been needed in a treatment trial.

To complicate matters further, before Francis took on trial oversight, Basil O'Connor had been busy promising communities that, if they participated, all second graders would be given vaccine. Under the scheme O'Connor was promoting, first and third graders would serve as *observed controls*. For Francis such a design was fatally flawed. There was too much opportunity for bias when everyone was aware of who received active vaccine and who did not. Unfortunately, it was by this time too late for the National Foundation to retreat from its promise. After much discussion, the observed control design continued and blinded, placebo control subjects were simply added to the trial.

To increase the chances that immunized children would be exposed to polio, Francis and his coinvestigators made the most of the descriptive epidemiologic data that had been catalogued for some years. The occurrence of disease varied in geography. Some counties across the country averaged annual rates of polio that were as much as 50% higher than most communities of similar size. In the 1952 epidemic, these places reported 58 polio cases per 100,000 in population compared with only 38 per 100,000 elsewhere. These high-rate communities became the logical locations in which to implement the trial.

Beginning April 1, 1954, first, second, and third graders in class-rooms across the United States rolled up their sleeves and subjected themselves to injections with either a cubic centimeter of Salk's for-malin-inactivated polio vaccine or a similar amount of colored water (see Figure 7-3). A sample of the children also had blood withdrawn so that any changes in antibody status could be determined. Over the ensuing weeks the children each received two more "shots" and gave more blood samples. Then everyone sat down to wait.

When the first cases of polio began to appear in early May, teams of evaluators went to work. This was a critical phase of the experiment. It was vital that every suspected case of polio was identified and examined. It was now that Francis's insistence on

FIGURE 7-3

Jonas Salk Administering Vaccine

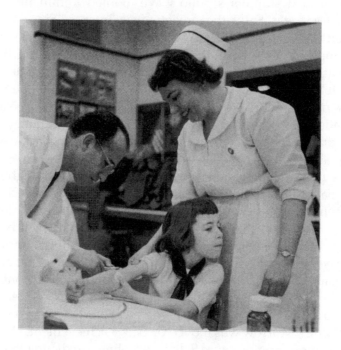

Source: March of Dimes Foundation.

the blinded placebo-controlled design mattered most. The bias he feared could easily arise if only "observed controls" were used: exaggerated reports of illness among those *not* receiving the "beneficial" injection and underreporting of disease among vaccine recipients. Francis was diligent to see that all field evaluators were rigorously trained in proper data collection. Requirements for reporting were clearly stated well in advance and definitions of what constituted polio were standardized. This phase of the trial lasted from May until the end of the following December. It then was time for Michigan's Evaluation Center to begin the painstaking process of compiling the data and producing the results.

Expectation was palpable. For O'Connor, who had invested over $7 million of the Foundation's money in the effort and plunged the organization into debt, the stakes were monumental. For millions of American parents, frantic for their children's future, the danger of next summer's polio wave loomed imminent. And, of course, for Jonas Salk, the anxiety was intense. Since the very beginning of the trial, Salk had fretted over the vaccine. He worried that some batches were not potent enough. He worried that the preservative that had been added was lessening the vaccine's activity. He felt harassed: by colleagues who demanded that he publish details of his work for professional audiences; by National Foundation publicists begging his assistance to raise money for the foundering foundation, and, of course, by reporters, each eager for a scoop about the miracle vaccine.

As pressure for public statements escalated throughout the winter, Salk found it more and more difficult to keep his desired distance from the press. Some relief came from an unexpected source, a newsman in whom Salk had found respect and trust: Edward R. Murrow. Host of a widely admired television news program called *See It Now*, Murrow had experienced polio firsthand. That summer his 8-year-old son, Casey, had suddenly complained of continuous aching in his legs and could not sit up. After a week of observation in the hospital, Casey was sent home recovered; he was one of the "lucky" ones. Murrow was moved by Salk's achievement. He understood the mounting pressure Salk was feeling, predicting that a successful trial would raise the latter to the state of "minor god." With only modest coaxing, Salk agreed to appear on *See It Now*. As the untutored scientist moved toward the brink of becoming a celebrity, Murrow took on the role of mentor. "Young man," the newsman counseled as they completed the broadcast, "a great tragedy has befallen you—you have lost your anonymity" (3, p. 402).

Finally, in early April 1955, Francis announced that the analysis was complete; a news conference to announce results was scheduled for April 12. The date was significant. It was the 10th anniversary of the day that polio's most celebrated victim, Franklin Roosevelt, had died. Some criticized the "rocket's red glare and flashbulbs bursting in air" atmosphere of the press conference (2, pp. 432–433). It was far from the standard scientific forum, where academics speak only to each other and quibble over every piece of data that is presented. This was a public event that the entire world was watching. Writers and photographers elbowed one another for prime positions for hours before the news conference began.

The news was good. The vaccine worked. In a 98-minute monologue, Francis detailed the findings (4). In the critical placebo-controlled arm, over 400,000 children had completed the immunizations and follow-up—about 200,000 in each group. There were 244 cases of polio reported altogether, 82 among vaccine recipients and 162 among placebo controls. These numbers translated into rates of 41 per 100,000 population and 81 per 100,000, respectively (see Table 7-1). Using the *ratio of these rates* to calculate an estimate of *risk*, placebo recipients were twice as likely to contract polio as those receiving vaccine (81/100,000 ÷ 41/100,000 = 2.0). Inverting the numbers (the reciprocal) states the case another way: A vaccinated child had only .51, or 51%, of the risk of getting poliomyelitis as a control child (41/100,000 ÷ 81/100,000 = .51).*

Such performance is reasonable but not outstanding. It is certainly far short of the 100% efficacy the newspapers had rumored or to which Salk aspired. But here, Francis's rigorous methods provided help. He had insisted on strict criteria for accepting cases of polio and not all reports ultimately met the standards. Almost 15% were relegated into "doubtful" or "not poliomyelitis" categories. These became *misclassified* cases. When they are subtracted from the count and only *confirmed* cases of polio included, the estimate of vaccine efficacy changes. Table 7-1 shows the results. The case count falls to 57 in the vaccination group and to 142 among placebo recipients; this means new rates of 28 per 100,000 and 71 per 100,000, respectively and a more favorable rate ratio of 2.5 to 1 (71/ 100,000 ÷ 28/100,000 = 2.5). Control subjects were 2.5 times more likely to contract polio than vaccinees; that means vaccinees experienced only 39% the rate of polio as controls. The vaccine reduced cases by 61% (1 − .39 × 100 = 61) or, is 61% *efficacious*. Performance clearly improves when only confirmed cases of polio are included in the analysis.

---

* This latter ratio can be used to calculate the percentage reduction in disease that is associated with the vaccine. Subtracting .51 from 1 (the *complement* of the ratio) gives the percent reduction attributable to vaccine: 49. This figure may also be thought of as the vaccine efficacy, its power to protect against the illness. Salk's vaccine reduced the rate of polio among recipients by 49%; it was 49% *efficacious*.

TABLE 7-1

Cases of Polio Among Vaccine and Placebo Recipients
with Risk and Efficacy Estimates Using Two Differing
Classifications of Cases

Experimental Group	Number of Subjects	Number of Cases	Rate Cases/ 100,000 Subjects	Risk Ratio b/a	Risk Ratio a/b	Efficacy (1 − a/b)
All Reported Cases						
Vaccine (a)	200,745	82	41			
Placebo (b)	201,229	162	81	2.0	0.51	0.49
Confirmed Polio Only						
Vaccine (a)	200,745	57	28			
Placebo (b)	201,229	142	71	2.5	0.39	0.61

Source: Based on Francis (4).

Misclassification of subjects is of critical concern in medical research. It occurs whenever subjects entering a study don't have the condition or disease in question, or are incorrectly determined to have the outcome that is sought. Results can be distorted and conclusions mistaken. Most often misclassification is *nondifferential*. This means that, as in the polio trial, subjects in both the active treatment and placebo arms are equally susceptible. Both groups had reported "cases" that were not confirmed as polio. The net effect of this is to dilute or lessen differences between the groups. Nondifferential misclassification tends to mask potential benefits. In the Francis trial, removing misclassified cases improved the estimate of vaccine efficacy; it rose from 50 to 61%.

Misclassification can also be *differential*, or *biased*. It was this type of error that Francis wished to exclude by insisting upon placebo controls and blinded assessment. When neither subjects nor evaluators know who receives active vaccine and who does not, tendencies (intentional or not) to minimize disease in active vaccines and overestimate it in nonrecipients are mitigated. The trial's careful design reduced the chance that any differences in rates of cases between the groups and subsequent estimates of vaccine benefit were due to bias.

The vaccine wasn't perfect. The trial had been mounted quickly and, as Salk had feared, there were some vaccine lots in which the potency was low. But with Salk's unfailing belief in the vaccine and its potential for improvement, the results were good enough. They were what the world needed. Rejoicing was widespread, in Salk's laboratory, in the offices of the National Foundation, among most scientists, and, of course, among the public. By the afternoon of April 12, a special vaccine advisory committee of the federal government had been convened to recommend that the vaccine be licensed for distribution to doctor's offices and health clinics across the land. There was still time to immunize the country's children against the approaching summer's epidemic.

In anticipation of a favorable report from Francis, vaccine manufacturers had already stockpiled supplies and were ready as soon as licensure was announced. Immunization programs began the day after the vaccine was proclaimed a success. "Victory" over polio seemed now at hand, and on April 22 Salk was summoned to the White House rose garden to receive the nation's thanks and a citation from President Dwight Eisenhower.

Three days later, it all started to unravel. On April 25, an infant who had been injected with polio vaccine was brought to Michael Reese Hospital in Chicago with both legs paralyzed. The following day, the California State Health Department acknowledged 5 reported cases of paralytic polio among children who had received vaccine only 4 to 10 days earlier. In each case, paralysis involved the arm in which the injection had been given. Fear grew throughout the country. Because the vaccine was not 100% effective, it was understood that some children would contract polio in spite of being vaccinated. But this appeared to be quite another matter. April was not yet polio season. It seemed these children had contracted polio *because* of the vaccine.

The specter of the ill-fated experiments of 1935 reappeared. The questions were immediate and urgent. If these cases were vaccine related, were they simply the tip of the iceberg? How many more cases could be expected? How many other children were in danger? Would the episode undo all the hopes and promise of the successful field trial?

All 6 cases had been associated with a single manufacturer, Cutter Laboratories in Berkeley, California. But no one knew whether the problem resided with Cutter alone or extended to others. Even though the information was incomplete, on April 27 the Surgeon General of the Public Health Service (PHS) asked Cutter Laboratories to recall all of its vaccine. The following day, he directed an Atlanta branch of the PHS, known as the Communicable Disease Center (or CDC), to establish a polio surveillance unit to thoroughly investigate the apparent outbreak. Meanwhile, new cases continued to surface. Although all appeared related to the Cutter product, anxiety was high enough that, on May 7, the entire immunization program was suspended and a plant-by-plant inspection of all vaccine manufacturing facilities was ordered.

Meanwhile, the newly formed polio surveillance unit of the CDC was already at work. Alexander Langmuir, a public health physician with experience in the "polio wars," directed the group. A seasoned investigator, Langmuir had, in 1942, provided laboratory evidence that confirmed that polio was widely spread by seemingly healthy carriers. Epidemiologists from Langmuir's unit, known as the Epidemic Intelligence Service, or EIS, were immediately dispatched to gather details on the putative outbreak of vaccine-associated polio. Their task was formidable. They were to track down each new case of polio and determine its source.

Pounding the city pavements and trekking dusty rural roads in search of the details of disease was "shoe leather epidemiology." The EIS investigators scoured the country, from health departments to hospitals to clinics and doctor's offices, gathering specifics of the outbreak. It was an effort reminiscent of Caverly, but on a far grander scale. Uncertainty remained whether these cases were simply vaccine failures that coincided with the start of another polio season or whether the vaccine itself was causing the disease. After all, hundreds of thousands of vaccinations had already been given by the end of April, and with a vaccine that was only 60% effective, some cases could be expected to occur simply by chance.

The CDC epidemiologists worked their drill. They detailed person, place, and time to characterize the outbreak, and they uncovered vital information. They found 260 cases that occurred across the country from the middle of April to the first weeks of July. The western states, particularly Idaho and California, were the worst affected.

One finding immediately stood out. Not all the cases were in children who had been vaccinated. Only 94 of the 260 cases had received immunizations. Perhaps the vaccine was not responsible after all. But as nonvaccinated cases were investigated, a revealing pattern emerged: 126 of the cases occurred in family members of vaccinated children; the remaining 40 were among people residing in communities where vaccine programs had been launched. When cases were grouped as "vaccinated," "family contact," or "community contact," and charted by date of onset, the pattern shown in Figure 7-4 appeared (5).

Vaccinated cases appeared first and peaked about the first week in May. That was when family contact cases began, with most appearing in the last three weeks in May. Community contact cases began in earnest after May 14. The pattern supports the existence of a vaccine problem. If the vaccine virus were not completely killed, so that active virus was still present, the sequence makes sense. Live virus was given to children and caused disease in some. Vaccinees then shed virus and transmitted it to family members and others in the community. The sequential peaks and the distribution of groups of cases correspond with the incubation period of polio.

Another feature of the timing of the outbreak also implicated the vaccine. Figure 7-5 compares the occurrence of cases in 5 western states for the spring of 1955 (bottom chart) to the typical number of reported cases for the prior years from 1950 through 1954 (top chart). The patterns are quite different. Usually, polio begins in April and case numbers don't increase much before June. In contrast, in the spring of 1955 a peak occurred in May then declined sharply by mid-June. It was an atypical pattern, best explained by vaccine-induced cases. This early peak was particularly striking in Idaho, where polio was rarely seen in April and May. In preceding years, no more than 11 cases had been reported for the 10 weeks, from April 17 through June 25. In the spring of 1955, there were 88 (5).

Acknowledging that some early polio would occur regardless of the immunization program, CDC investigators calculated the number that would have been expected among vaccinees based on rates for previous years. Using data from school clinics in the western states for the critical period from April 17 to May 15, they determined that 10 cases were to be expected. In fact, there were 43 observed: an *observed-to-expected ratio* of 4 to 1. This comparison of *observed to*

FIGURE 7-4

Cutter Vaccine-Associated Cases by Week of Onset, 1955
(P = paralytic, NP = nonparalytic)

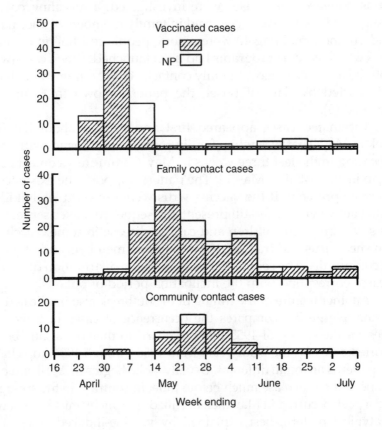

Source: From Nathanson & Langmuir (5).

expected is a useful concept. It requires knowing historic rates or rates in a larger population and applying them to a particular subgroup of interest. In this instance, the subgroup is the vaccinated children (just over 300,000) and the rate applied is the historic polio incidence among 6- to 8-year-olds from 1952.

The observed-to-expected ratio was also used to confirm the source of faulty vaccine. Five manufacturers contributed vaccine to the initial program effort. Cutter Laboratories actually had the smallest

FIGURE 7-5

Cutter Vaccine-Associated Cases by Onset, 1955 Compared
with Springtime Trend of Polio Incidence, 1950–1954 for
5 Western States

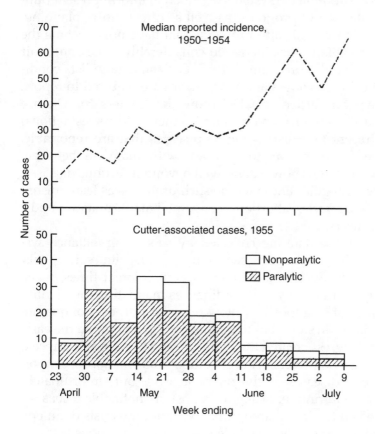

Source: From Nathanson & Langmuir (5).

share—about 300,000 vaccinations, just over 6% of the total. If cases
had been distributed proportionately among all the manufacturers,
8 cases would have been *expected* among Cutter recipients during the
initial campaign month. The number *observed* was *41*, a 5-to-1 ratio that
clearly implicated their product.

The intensive *surveillance* program begun at the time of the
"Cutter incident" is now regarded as an essential public health tool.

The elements of good surveillance consist of (1) a systematic approach to gathering accurate data, (2) the capacity to analyze and interpret the information, and (3) timely dissemination of the results. Good surveillance systems do much to inform present public health policies and programs as well as direct future planning. The number of public health problems that have now become the subject of surveillance has increased considerably since Langmuir established the polio program in 1955. Each state now lists conditions that health providers and laboratories are required to report. The data are forwarded to CDC (now the Centers for Disease Control and Prevention) which compiles them and issues national reports. A recent tally lists some 55 diseases that are reportable. They range from anthrax to typhoid, with many in between. Surveillance activities now extend well beyond infectious diseases. State and federal guidelines include such problems as lead poisoning, workplace injuries, abortions, congenital malformations, and a variety of cancers.

Most of these data are collected by *passive* surveillance systems. These rely upon reports sent in by doctors, clinics, hospitals, and laboratories. Such efforts have roots in colonial times, when towns would periodically issue ordinances mandating the identification of cases of smallpox or yellow fever for purposes of quarantine. Surveillance systems became more comprehensive in the early 1900s after Congress created the Public Health Service and directed the surgeon general to collect and compile information on important infectious diseases at the national level. But unfortunately, despite laws requiring reporting for a host of "notifiable diseases," compliance is often less than optimal. Without the crisis of an epidemic as an incentive, the task falls low on most priorities lists.

More aggressive, *active* surveillance, as was practiced following the polio field trials, provides more satisfactory results. Directed inquiries and an ongoing search for cases made through surveys, telephone calls, or personal visits, improve the quality of information. When a group of public health researchers compared results from routine passive reporting with active methods of mail solicitation and telephone contact, they found that mailed requests more than doubled and the telephone more than quadrupled reporting (6).

Active reporting is, of course, more labor intensive and, consequently, more costly than passive systems. A compromise is offered by the use of *sentinel systems,* in which a sample of health care providers is recruited to identify specific conditions such as automobile injuries or influenza. Their reports can provide timely information about disease trends or emerging health problems.

A number of ongoing national surveys sponsored by the National Center for Health Statistics complement surveillance activities. These carefully designed programs sample a variety of health-related issues, from the frequency of visits to doctor's offices to the average length of stay of nursing home patients, to the amount of zinc consumed in the typical American diet. Some surveys include measurement capabilities and can tell us how many children have too much lead in their blood, the average bone density of women over the age of 65, or the dimensions of the current epidemic of obesity.

Vaccine for all the manufacturers, except that of Cutter Laboratories, was cleared for rerelease by June 1. No further cases of vaccine-associated paralysis had occurred. Unfortunately, by then, the momentum that had followed the triumphant April announcement had been lost. It was autumn before the confidence of doctors and the public was reestablished, and immunizations resumed. By November there was evidence of progress. Langmuir reported that surveillance from 11 states and New York City indicated that children in the targeted age groups (5 to 10 years) had received more than 2.3 million doses of vaccine, with only 75 reported cases of paralytic polio. That was a rate of only 3.2 cases per 100,000 population. In contrast, unimmunized children of the same age groups had a rate of 13.2 per 100,000, a fourfold ratio (7). No further cases were attributed to the vaccine itself.

By 1961, over 400 million doses of Salk's inactivated virus had been given without further serious adverse events and cases of polio had plummeted. Rates had fallen from an average of 14.6 per 100,000 in the 5 years prior to licensing, to 1.8 per 100,000 in the postvaccine period; the reduction was almost 88%. Even a crusty epidemiologist like Langmuir, who never would attribute cause without sufficient evidence, admitted that "this reduction very substantially, if not entirely, can be attributed to the polio vaccine program"(8).

The year 1961 also saw the entrance of a rival to the Salk vaccine. A new, attenuated virus product was introduced.

This weakened strain of virus was, like Pasteur's rabies virus, made less virulent by repeated passage through tissue cultures. The resulting virus could stimulate immunity but did not cause disease. It was the work of Albert Sabin. He had caught up with Salk. Sabin's attenuated vaccine had several clear advantages over Salk's inactivated product. To begin with, it produced better immunity. Killed vaccine required a primary series of four doses, and annual boosters were recommended, if protection was to be maintained. Even with this rather daunting series of injections, levels of immunity still only reached 90%. The new vaccine also required multiple doses initially, but the resulting immunity appeared to last much longer. Another virtue, praised particularly by recipients, was that Sabin's vaccine was given by mouth. That meant no more painful shots. The oral-gastrointestinal route, which mirrors polio's natural pathway of infection, also meant the living virus was similarly excreted. So vaccine virus, like its "wild" cousin, spread to family members and other close contacts. Following infection, contacts then became immune as well. It is an added benefit—for the most part. There was, unfortunately, one serious drawback. Occasionally, the attenuated virus *reverted* to its more dangerous form. A small number of individuals, particularly those with compromised immune systems, cancer patients on chemotherapy or those with immune-deficient diseases, came down with polio, often with serious, even fatal consequences.

Following its introduction, Sabin vaccine became the standard, and, as it was generally deployed, rates of polio continued to decline. By 1965, just 10 years after Salk's vaccine first came available, only 61 paralytic cases occurred in the United States. The year 1979 marked the last one in which naturally occurring polio was reported in this country. From 1980 through 1989, reports of cases continued—averaging about 8 per year. A handful of these were "imported," brought in from outside the country; but 95% were due to the vaccine. The point had been reached, as earlier with smallpox vaccination, where the vaccine posed a greater risk than the disease. In 1999, it was decided to abandon the highly successful Sabin oral vaccine and return to an inactivated virus that would neither multiply nor spread. No vaccine-associated cases have been reported since then.

The success in eliminating polio in the United States (and in many western European countries) raised hopes for worldwide eradication. In 1985, the Pan American Health Organization (PAHO) announced that it would rid the Western Hemisphere of polio by 1990. The PAHO program featured national immunization days, in which millions of children were immunized on massive single-day events. But the program also depended to a great extent on an active surveillance program to track down cases and immunize communities where they occurred. PAHO missed its target only by a year. In 1991, a wild virus-associated case from Peru became the last in the Western Hemisphere.

The World Health Organization (WHO) also took on the challenge. Their goal was global eradication of the virus by the year 2000. While this objective is not yet in hand, we are closing in. In 2002, the number of polio-endemic countries fell to 7, the lowest ever. Even within these nations, located in Africa and the Indian subcontinent, the occurrence of disease is geographically restricted. In fact, 99% of the 1900 cases reported in the world were found in India, Nigeria, and Pakistan. And 80% of these were limited to only 6 of the 76 states or provinces of these 3 countries (9).

It is a remarkable story. In little more than 100 years the life cycle of an epidemic has almost been completed: from first delineation of the problem, to identification of its cause, to creation and deployment of preventive measures. Poliomyelitis is on the edge of extinction. Wouldn't Charles Caverly have been pleased?

REFERENCES

1. *Infantile Paralysis in Vermont, 1894–1922; A Memorial to Charles S. Caverly, M.D.* Burlington, Vermont: State Department of Public Health; 1924.
2. Paul JR. *A History of Poliomyelitis.* New Haven: Yale University Press; 1971.
3. Persico JE. *Edward R. Murrow: An American Original.* New York: McGraw-Hill; 1988.
4. Francis T, Jr., Korns RF, Voight RB, et al. An evaluation of the 1954 poliomyelitis vaccine trials. *Am J Public Health.* May 1955; 45(5, Part 2):1–63.

5. Nathanson N, Langmuir A. The Cutter incident: poliomyelitis following formaldehyde-inactivated poliovirus vaccination in the United States during the spring of 1955, Part II. Relationship of poliomyelitis to Cutter vaccine. *Am J Hyg.* 1963; 78:29–59.

6. Thacker SB, Redmond S, Rothenberg RB, Spitz SB, Choi KC, White MC. A controlled trial of disease surveillance strategies. *Am J Prev Med.* 1986; 2:345–350.

7. Langmuir A, Nathanson N, Jackson Hall W. Surveillance of poliomyelitis in the United States in 1955. *AJPH.* 1956; 46:75–88.

8. Langmuir A. The surveillance of communicable diseases of national importance. *N Engl J Med.* 1963; 268:182–191.

9. *Global Polio Eradication Initiative: Progress 2002.* Geneva: World Health Organization; 2003.

A Cancer Grows: Edward R. Murrow and the Cigarette

When Jonas Salk spoke of Edward R. Murrow (see Figure 8-1), his tone was one of reverence:

> He was instantly a remarkable human being to me. You could see the depth of his soul, in a sense through his eyes. He could draw out the essence of one's life....I felt, in a spiritual sense, that I had met my match. I found him introspective, meditative, with a purity of thought. He had true pitch. He was someone who in another age might have been a mystic. To me, Ed was a teacher, a preacher, a minister, a guide, but a teacher especially, in the best sense of the word, helping others to understand so they might make better choices. (1, p. 402)

Murrow had coached Salk through the latter's most trying moments of 1955, just prior to the announcement of the polio vaccine trial results. Ten years later, it was Salk's turn to reciprocate. But when Murrow arrived in beautiful La Jolla, California, at Salk's newly formed Institute for Biologic Studies, there was little of the man who had inspired Salk. Ed Murrow was dying of lung cancer.

Since the 1930s Murrow had been the dean of broadcast journalism, his name synonymous with intellect, integrity, and plain-spoken eloquence. Murrow first earned acclaim through a stunning series of broadcast firsts. In the terrifying nights of the 1940 Nazi blitzkrieg on London, he risked himself on the city's rooftops to

FIGURE 8-1

Edward R. Murrow

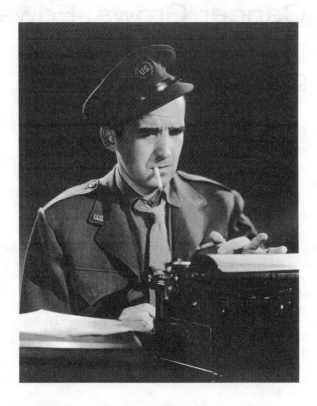

Source: Edward R. Murrow Collection, Digital Collections and Archives, Tufts University.

transmit eyewitness accounts of the attacks. His familiar baritone riveted Americans to their radios, painting verbal pictures of the incendiaries illuminating the English sky. Later he accompanied bombers in raids over Germany and was one of the first reporters to enter the concentration camps.

Following the war, Murrow transferred his talents to the nascent world of television news. In 1951, he launched a program on the Columbia Broadcasting System (CBS), called *See It Now*. It featured detailed reporting and in-depth analyses on trenchant social and political issues of the day. During the 7 years the program ran, Murrow took on such provocative subjects as life on the front lines of the Korean War, school segregation in the south, and book burning in California, as well as the 2 exclusive interviews with the creator of the Salk vaccine. Though his was a serious voice, that continually prodded Americans to self-examination, Murrow also had a self-deprecating humor that helped him keep perspective. He once remarked to Salk, when the 2 were riding in a cab to Murrow's studio: "I'm off to poison the minds of the people" (1, p. 402). And on another occasion was heard to say, "Just because your voice reaches halfway around the world doesn't mean you are wiser than when it reached only to the end of the bar."

Of all Murrow's *See It Now* broadcasts, the one for which he is most remembered was his prime-time exposé of Wisconsin's anti-communist crusader, Senator Joseph McCarthy. By the spring of 1954 when the program aired, McCarthy and his Committee on Un-American Activities had paralyzed the country's conscience. Allegations of communist conspiracies were flying; reputations lay in ruins; careers were crushed; and artists and intellectuals fled to Europe in numbers. Men in the nation's highest offices were dumb in fear of McCarthy's rage. But the senator's bullying methods struck at Murrow's soul. They violated his profound belief in our treasured freedoms. Knowing there was sure to be retaliation, Murrow crafted a documentary that, by simply splicing samples of the senator's behavior, revealed the politician's malice and mendacity to the entire nation. It was an awakening. Finally, America stirred. McCarthy mounted the predicted counterattack, but his efforts to discredit Murrow failed. *See It Now* marked the beginning of demagogue McCarthy's decline.

Another controversy, to which See It Now devoted several episodes, was news of a link between cigarette smoking and lung cancer. By the middle 1950s, increasing bits of medical research were pointing toward tobacco as responsible for a rising number of cancer cases. Some scientists and, not surprisingly, the tobacco industry shrugged off the evidence as inconclusive. Murrow's programs presented both sides of the debate, but he himself was skeptical. But then, his reservations about the connection between smoking and cancer might have been influenced by his own addiction. Smoking typically from 60 to 80 cigarettes a day, Murrow admitted to grave doubts that he could "spend a half hour without a cigarette with any comfort or ease" (2, p. 497). He did refrain from smoking on camera during the *See It Now* programs on tobacco, but on most public occasions, including his usual television appearances, a cigarette was invariably in hand.

His habit survived all evidence and efforts to quell it. He was undeterred by the chronic bronchitis of his son, Casey, which persisted throughout the child's years in the Murrow's smoke-filled home. He was not persuaded by his own racking fits of coughing that so unsettled friends they feared he was expiring before their eyes. The removal of a cancerous lung from his similarly addicted brother was not enough; nor was Salk's offer to show him photographs of smokers' lungs. Nothing stopped him.

By the fall of 1963, Murrow had grown disillusioned with network television—its pandering to the whims of sponsors, the fear of controversy, the absence of integrity. His open criticism of the industry produced a rift with CBS and estranged him from a number of his broadcast colleagues. When asked by the country's new president, John Kennedy, to head the U.S. Information Agency, Murrow agreed. The new job was demanding. In Murrow's first 18 months at the agency, he lost 8 pounds from a frame that was already lean. In late September, while on a demanding tour to Philadelphia with endless interviews and speeches, his voice broke down. His throat hurt and he could scarcely speak. He immediately returned to Washington and checked into a hospital. His problem, it turned out, was more than one of simple overwork. On October 6, in a 3-hour operation, doctors removed a cancerous left lung.

To a man of Murrow's temperament, it was a devastating blow. To demonstrate his self-control, he banished smoking. But it was a futile gesture. In the end, it only added to growing anxiety and depression. His energy was drained from radiation treatments that followed surgery and the loss of half his lung capacity. The January 1964 visit to Salk's Institute in southern California was meant to cheer Murrow with sunshine, golf, and the stimulation of the institute's collected intellectuals. But the weather was foul, cold and wet; the golf was too tiring; and Murrow sequestered himself in the cliffside house Salk had found for him. The effort was not a success. After 3 months, Murrow returned to the east, where he patched a few relationships with broadcast colleagues and participated in a final reminiscence on the history of CBS radio. But the path was downward. By November, the cancer had spread to his brain, and on April 27, 1965, he died, two days past his 57th birthday.

The disease that took the life of Edward Murrow is different from many of the maladies we have seen before. It does not come as an onslaught of multiplying microbes that stirs a great inflammatory response and is concluded within weeks in either recovery or demise. Cancer is a slow and insidious affair. It is a *chronic* disease, at work for months, or more often, years. Nor is it a single entity, but rather a designation that includes a collection of kindred diseases affecting various body sites and types of cells. All share the common feature of abnormal, unregulated cell growth, but cancers have different patterns of growth and spread, and different causes. They can afflict the brain, the blood, the breast, or the bowel. They can grow rapidly and spread aggressively in months or smolder in a single site for many years. They can be the result of a genetic predisposition, a personal habit, or exposure to an environmental agent.

Cancer strikes at the soul of the cell, at the genes that program and regulate the cell's most basic functions. Cancers arise from mutations, from damage to the genes that manage processes that make our vital proteins and control cell reproduction. These mutations can occur spontaneously or be triggered by external agents such as chemical compounds or radiation. Fortunately, the body has systems to repair such damage, usually by eliminating defective cells before they reproduce themselves. Occasionally, repair programs themselves become defective, and mutant cells within a tissue like the breast or bowel are allowed to reproduce. Unchecked, these abnormal cells grow into tumors, aberrant tissue that is without healthy purpose. The worst of these abnormal growths, characterized as *malignant*, can grow rapidly, displacing healthy cells and spreading or *metastasizing* through the body by the blood or lymphatic systems.

Edward Murrow's cancer came from cells that line the airways of the lung, the trachea, and bronchi. His cancer is a 20th-century phenomenon. It was rarely seen before the 1930s. But by the early 1960s, when Murrow was diagnosed, the disease had grown epidemic. In only 30 years, deaths in men from lung cancer had surged from 1800 in 1930 to over 40,000 in the year that Murrow died. What was the cause of this remarkable increase? What had happened in the brief span of 30 years that might account for such a dramatic rise? The nature of the lesion, a growth deep within the lung, suggested that something toxic was inhaled. Some thought it could be related to the massive outbreaks of influenza of several decades earlier.

Some thought it due to growing levels of industrial pollution. Automobiles in particular were suspected. But another, respiratory exposure for which there was a well-documented increase, was that of cigarette smoking.

It surprises many that although tobacco has been used in America since before Columbus found natives smoking pipes, cigarette smoking is a relatively recent habit. Consumption data from the U.S. Department of Agriculture (shown in Table 8-1) reveal that in 1900 annual per person use of tobacco products included only 49 cigarettes, compared with 111 cigars, 1.6 pounds of pipe tobacco, and 0.1 pounds of chewing tobacco. By 1960, use of the latter 3 had fallen 2-fold to 8-fold. By contrast, cigarette smoking had increased 8000%, to an average per-person consumption of almost 4000 per year. When the increases in cigarette consumption and lung cancer deaths are placed together in a single graph, as in Figure 8-2, the association between the two factors is striking. Of note is the lag between increased consumption (beginning about 1930) and the rise in lung cancer deaths, which begins after 1950. This interval of approximately 20 years suggests a latent period during which cancer develops.

TABLE 8-1

Annual Consumption of Tobacco Products Per Person
15 Years Old and Over, 1900–1960

Year	Cigarettes (Number)	Cigars (Number)	Pipe Tobacco (Pounds)	Chewing Tobacco (Pounds)
1900	49	111	1.6	4.1
1910	138	113	2.6	3.9
1920	611	117	2.0	3.1
1930	1365	72	1.9	1.9
1940	1828	56	2.1	1.0
1950	3322	50	.9	.8
1960	3888	57	.6	.5

Source: From: Smoking & Health (3).

FIGURE 8-2

Cigarette Consumption (in billions) and Number of Deaths from Lung Cancer, United States, 1900–990

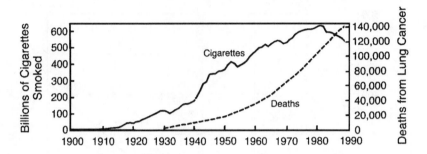

Source: Smoking tobacco and cancer program (4).

A similar relationship is seen in Figure 8-3. Here, cigarette consumption on a country-by-country basis is compared with lung cancer mortality rates that occur 20 years later. Again, there seems clear relationship between cigarette consumption and lung cancer.

A bit of caution in interpretation is required here, however. The data shown in these two figures are *ecological* in nature. That means that they describe groups (whole years or whole countries) rather than individuals. We know that lung cancer in the aggregate increases relative to growing cigarette consumption. But the data don't provide the details whether the people who actually consumed cigarettes were the ones who contracted cancer. The relationship is plausible (especially with our present knowledge), but it is possible that smoking rates are simply a marker or surrogate for some other factor that is the real culprit. Other environmental factors may have changed over the same time that rates of cigarette smoking grew. Industrial air pollution and auto emissions, for example, also increased during this interval. These, rather than tobacco smoke, could be responsible for the lung cancer rise.

A more accurate picture of the relationship between lung cancer and smoking requires data that correlate disease and exposure at an individual's level. Beginning in 1950, such evidence began to appear.

FIGURE 8-3

Cigarette Consumption (per capita) in 1930 and Death Rates in Males (per million) in Various Countries in 1950

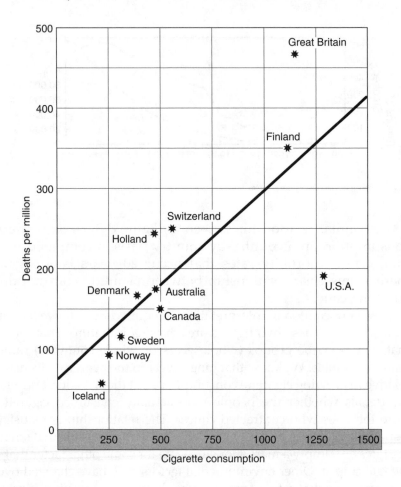

Source: Doll (5).

At the Barnes Hospital in St. Louis, two researchers, named Ernst L. Wynder and Evarts Graham, had been interested in lung cancer for some time. The two had been participants on Murrow's programs on cigarettes and lung cancer. Graham was a respected surgeon, the first to successfully remove a human lung. He had watched his number of lung cancer patients grow for 20 years. Wynder was his student. For a summer project Wynder had begun interviewing lung cancer patients about their smoking habits. The two men continued gathering data until they had information on more than 600 lung cancer cases (6).

Their collection came from hospitals and physician practices across the United States, from California to Massachusetts. To be certain that the reports collected were, in fact, due to lung cancer, the investigators obtained and reviewed pathologic specimens from each patient, verifying under the microscope that lung cancer cells were present. Because hospital records rarely supply the detailed personal information they sought, Wynder and Graham obtained specific information on every patient by personal interviews (or in a small number of instances, mailed questionnaires). "What lung diseases have you had? Do you smoke? How much? What tobacco products do you use? For how long? When did you begin to smoke? Do you inhale?" The questionnaire included occupational histories to identify possible exposures to dusts or fumes, as well as places of residence, education, use of alcohol, and causes of death of family members.

In all, 630 cases of documented cancer of the lung were assembled. Of these, 605 were in men and only 25 in women (a ratio of 24 to 1). Such imbalance of males and females raised the question whether the disease was likely to be similar in men and women. So Wynder and Graham restricted their analysis to the largest group, the men. Lung cancer patients ranged in age from early 30s to the late 70s, but the large proportion was in the 50- to 70-year-old age range. Only 2.3% of cases were under 40. Almost all smoked. In fact, only 1.3% of the more than 600 men reported that they used no tobacco. Over 90% smoked cigarettes, and 99% of these admitted they inhaled. Moreover, the smoking had gone on for many years. In fact, 96% of subjects had smoked for 20 years or more and 85% for more than 30 years. When the amount each man smoked was categorized from "light" (1 to 9 cigarettes per day for greater than 20 years) to "chain" (35+ cigarettes per day for 20 years or more), with intermediate classifications of "moderately heavy" (10 to 15 per day) to "heavy" (16 to 20 per day) to "excessive" (21 to 34 per day), it was discovered that 86% of patients were in the "heavy" smoking category or higher.

These data by themselves seem potent evidence to build a case. But Wynder and Graham recognized the need for a comparison group. Though the exposure to cigarette smoking in their cancer patients was very high, overall consumption of tobacco in the country was substantial. The smoking habits of lung cancer patients might simply reflect high levels in society at large. An estimate was needed of patterns of cigarette use among American men who didn't have lung cancer. Accordingly, the questionnaire on smoking habits was administered to 780 male patients on the medical and surgical wards of the St. Louis hospitals who were without the disease. When smoking patterns for cancer patients were compared with these control subjects, the results in Figure 8-4 appear. Indeed, smoking among control patients was high; fewer than 15% were nonsmokers. Yet the distribution of amounts smoked between the groups differed noticeably. Results showed that 51% of cancer of patients smoked a pack a day of cigarettes or more for 20 years. Only 19% of control subjects did so.

Although this magnitude of difference may not seem great, the calculated risk is actually substantial. Among the 605 lung cancer cases, 592 smoked cigarettes and only 8 did not. That proportion compares with 666 smokers and 114 nonsmokers among the 780 control subjects. We can estimate risk by making a comparison between the *odds* of smoking among lung cancer cases with the similar odds among controls. The odds of smoking among lung

FIGURE 8-4

Percentages of Amount of Smoking Among 605 Male Patients with Lung Cancer (solid bars) and 780 Hospitalized Men without Lung Cancer (lined bars)

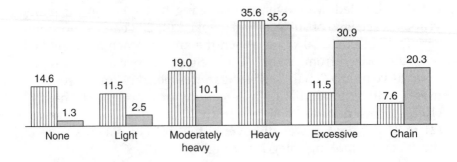

Source: Wynder & Graham (6, pp. 329–336).

cancer cases are 597 to 8, or 75 to 1; 75 cases of lung cancer smoke for every 1 who doesn't. This compares with odds of 5.8 to 1 (666 smokers to 114 nonsmokers) among controls. Comparison of these two sets of odds, 75 to 1 over 5.8 to 1, produces an *odds* ratio of 12.9. In plainer prose, it means that lung cancer patients are almost 13 times more likely than controls to smoke cigarettes.* A 13-fold ratio is very high.

The same issue of the *Journal of the American Medical Association* that published Wynder and Graham's findings contained a 2nd report on smoking and cancer. It was by a group from the New York State Health Department (7). Investigators Mortin Levin, Hyman Goldstein, and Paul Gerhardt took an approach that varied somewhat from that of the St. Louis research team. Their cancer patients came from a single hospital, a cancer center in the Buffalo area called Roswell Park. Because of its specialty nature, patients admitted there were strongly suspected of having cancer, though the diagnosis was not always confirmed. In fact, at the time of the study, approximately 50% of admissions turned out *not* to have a malignancy. These patients formed the comparison group. A particular boon to the study was the long-standing practice at Roswell Park of obtaining detailed information on patients' habits upon admission. Included was detailed information on smoking habits.

The researchers identified 1045 male cancer patients, 236 of whom had lung cancer. Other cancer sites were also in the study, including cancers of the throat, esophagus, and rectum. There were 605 men who were ultimately found to be free of cancer who became controls. As Table 8-2 reveals, 66% of lung cancer patients smoked cigarettes. This frequency fell to 48% for other cancer patients and to 44% for patients without cancer. Again, the accusing finger wagged at cigarettes.

The research approach used in both these studies is known as the *case-control* design. Investigators begin by identifying persons with a particular disease, then explore their past, seeking information on exposures or behaviors that might be precursors to the problem.

---

* The odds ratio provides an estimate of the risk that a smoker will develop lung cancer. Odds ratios approximate the risk ratios that we have seen before, though saying that lung cancer patients are more likely to be smokers and that smokers are more likely to get lung cancer is not quite the same.

TABLE 8-2

Prevalence of Cigarette Smokers by Diagnostic Category
for 1507 Patients in Roswell Park Cancer Center

Diagnosis	No. Cases	Percentage Smokers
Lung cancer	236	66.1
Other cancer	666	48.0
Lung disease (non-tumors)	124	53.1
Other noncancer	481	44.1

Source: Based on Levin et al. (7).

Exposure can be to a wide variety of "agents"—asbestos or coal dust, pesticides or radioactivity, a high-fat diet or low exercise, hormone replacements or immunization against measles, or tobacco smoke. Exposures may be "excessive" in the case of a toxin, such as lead or Agent Orange, or "too little," as with a vitamin or other essential nutrient. Critical to the determination is, of course, the presence of a comparison group, a group that gauges the expected or usual exposure.

The case-control design is high on efficiency. It is relatively easy to identify cases of a disease in hospitals, clinics, or physician offices. Once found, cases are usually receptive to discussing past habits or exposures that may illuminate the source of their disease. Because exposures have occurred in the past and disease is current, there is no wait required to determine outcomes. The data are available in present time.

The case-control design has challenges as well. These are nicely illustrated in the early studies on tobacco. To begin with, it should be clear that a proper choice of cases is required. Selected subjects must have the disease in question—in the present analysis, lung cancer. As we discovered when classifying polio in Chapter 7, including as cases individuals without disease obscures results. If patients with lung cancer are in fact heavier smokers, then adding non–lung cancer patients (such as those with lesions from tuberculosis) to the pool is likely to dilute results. The added subjects will, in all probability, smoke at a lower, general population rate and mask the difference between cases and controls. Mindful of this problem, Wynder and Graham required pathologic confirmation of the cancer diagnosis before a case was included in their study. This is sound practice though not always feasible.

Finally, it's essential that cases are not chosen *because* they have a history of exposure to the risk in question. The toxic shock syndrome (TSS) that was epidemic in the early 1980s presents a case in point. The illness usually struck women of reproductive age with sudden onset of high fever, rash, and falling blood pressure, sometimes with life-threatening shock. But the disease had not been seen before, and its diagnosis was not always clear. As researchers were recruiting subjects for a case-control investigation to elucidate its cause, suspicions were already abroad that TSS afflicted only menstruating women who were using tampons. Because fever and rash are signs common to many diseases, the information that a patient was also using tampons might tip an undecided doctor toward the diagnosis of TSS. If the presence of the risk factor *leads* to selection as a case, results will be biased. Cases will be far more likely than controls to have a history of tampon use.*

Identifying appropriate control subjects is also essential. The purpose of the comparison group is to establish a background or prevalent level of risk or exposure within the population from which cases are derived. What is the pattern of tobacco use among middle-aged American men (the source of lung cancer cases) in the middle 1900s? Do smoking patterns among lung cancer cases differ from this? If the comparison group does not reflect the typical prevalence of risk or exposure, then estimates of association will not be correct. In general, control subjects should have characteristics that are similar to cases (for example, age group, race, sex, marital and socioeconomic status). The obvious difference is the absence of the disease in question. Several options are available to investigators in choosing controls. As with cases, hospitals and other medical facilities are good sources for comparison subjects. Individuals are readily available, are frequently from the same community, and also share the common experience of being in the hospital for a medical problem.

---

* Concerns over bias were addressed when investigators analyzed their findings, and tampon use
  was still found to be strongly associated with TSS.

Wynder and Graham recruited control subjects from local hospitals, where they could be conveniently and efficiently interviewed. So did Levin and colleagues. But are these hospitalized patients the best controls? Do they give accurate estimates of smoking habits of the population that produced the cases of lung cancer? The shared experience of hospitalization may make controls desirable, but it can also create a problem. If the diseases that prompted the hospitalization of non–lung cancer patients are related to cigarette smoking, then the comparison may be flawed. We know, for example, that smoking brings on other lung diseases like emphysema and bronchitis. If such patients become control subjects, then the frequency of smoking among controls will be higher than that in the general population. Any difference between cases and controls will be diminished and the association between smoking and lung cancer blunted.

Levin's data, displayed in Table 8-2, support this. The highest frequency of smokers among the 4 groups being compared is in lung cancer patients. Second highest is among subjects with other lung disease, and the lowest is among patients without cancer or other lung disease. The magnitude of the association between lung cancer and smoking depends on which of the comparison groups one chooses. The relationship will be highest when noncancer, non–lung disease subjects are used and less if patients with other lung diseases become controls. Because hospitalized patients are *selectively* admitted on the basis of tobacco-related illnesses, they bias the study's findings.

Concern that hospitalized patients may have diseases that confuse the picture often prompts investigators to look for controls outside of hospitals or doctor's offices. The communities that produced the cases are often a better option. *Neighborhood* or *friend controls* of the same age and sex are likely to be of similar socioeconomic background and may share other similarities with cases. Such controls can often be identified by subjects themselves or found by house-to-house surveys. It should, however, be noted that friends and neighbors may share more than social class and proximity with cases. If they also have similar habits such as smoking, then relating these to cause becomes a problem.

Another approach is the telephone survey. Potential controls are identified from phone books, voter lists, or other community rosters.

Alternatively, controls may be contacted by a process known as *random digit dialing*, where a particular telephone area code and exchange (the first 3 digits) are matched to those of cases and the final 4 numbers chosen by a random process. Although many randomly dialed calls are needed to produce a suitable comparison group, the resulting controls usually represent a cross-section of the community. Of course, one needs to have a telephone or be registered to vote to make it to the list. And that qualification excludes some folks from being controls.

Once selections have been made, researchers hope that cases and controls are similar. Unfortunately, they not always are. After selecting their controls, Wynder and Graham realized that their 2 groups differed in some important respects. More of the cases were concentrated in the older age brackets than controls (see Table 8-3). Wynder and Graham worried that this difference in age distribution could influence their findings, if age were related both to smoking and to development of lung cancer. In fact, such is the case. Older subjects are more likely to have lung cancer but are less likely to be cigarette smokers. Comparisons could be confused by the differing age distributions. Controls, being younger and heavier smokers, don't properly represent the population from which the cases come. They are likely to produce an inflated estimate of general smoking prevalence and to underestimate the smoking differences between the groups.

In epidemiologic terms, this represents a *confounded* situation. Age is related to both the exposure (smoking) and the outcome (lung cancer).

TABLE 8-3

Distribution and Prevalence of Cigarette Smoking by Age Group for 605 Male Lung Cancer Cases and 780 Controls

	Age Distribution		*Percent Smokers*	
Age Group	**Cases**	**Controls**	**Cases**	**Controls**
30–49 years	19.7	39.7	90.7	62.6
50–59 years	42.6	26.9	89.5	60.5
60–79 years	37.7	33.3	79.8	44.2

Source: Based on Wynder & Graham (6).

It's the same type of problem we encountered in Chapter 5, with mortality and age distributions in Alaska and Florida. If the influence of age were equalized across the two groups, the relationship of smoking to lung cancer would be clarified. The approach is to compare the frequency of smoking among cases and controls within similar age groups, in the 30- to 49-year-olds, in the 50- to 59-year-olds, and so on. Then any differences in age distributions are neutralized.

The right-hand side of Table 8-3 shows that the frequency of heavy smoking (a pack a day or more) decreases among the older ages, for both cases and controls. But it also shows that cases smoke more heavily across all three categories of age. This is a *stratified analysis*. It *controls* the problem of confounding by age. It does not, alas, produce a convenient composite estimate of the frequency of smoking within the groups of cases and controls. Again, as in Chapter 5, a summary or *adjusted* smoking prevalence for each group can be calculated by applying the *age-specific* percentages of smokers to the age distribution of a single, *standard population*. This may be a general population of the region or country or, as in the case of Wynder and Graham's study, the combined group of cases and controls. The *age-adjusted* frequencies of smoking are, in fact, the numbers that both Wynder and Graham and Levin and colleagues present in their reports.

Confounding by age is a common bane of health research. Many diseases increase in frequency with age (for example, heart disease, high blood pressure, diabetes) as do risks of some habits or exposures (for example, increasing weight, low exercise, poor vitamin intake). But age confounding is only one example. Any time a disease outcome relates to more than one risk or exposure and the exposures are associated, confusion awaits.

Another type of cancer illustrates the point. Cancer of the mouth and throat occurs more frequently in heavy users of tobacco. But an association with alcohol has also been observed. Because the habits of smoking and drinking often go together, it is possible that only one of the agents is actually causal and the other is confounding—along for the ride.

Researchers examined these relationships among a group of Veterans Administration hospital patients in New York City (8). Their case-control study compared the histories of smoking and alcohol consumption for 598 men with mouth or throat cancer with

598 controls. Results are shown in Table 8-4. This table combines the data to display not frequencies, as we have seen before, but relative risk for each level of exposure. For subjects who don't smoke or drink the risk of oral cancer is 1.0, the baseline value. Reading across the table rows yields cancer risks for a given level of alcohol consumption as smoking increases. For nondrinkers, the risk grows from 1.0 to 2.4. The columns provide risk estimates for increasing alcohol use when level of smoking is held constant. Nonsmokers experience a rising risk from 1.0 to 2.3 when they drink 1.6 ounces of alcohol or more each day. The table helps clarify the question whether alcohol or smoking is the factor associated with oral cancer. They both are. For each level of tobacco use, increased drinking raises the risk of cancer. The same is true for alcohol. The association between alcohol and oral cancer is not an artifact of confounding by smoking, nor vice-versa.

A researcher's ability to control confounding factors by analyzing results among similar subgroups (age, sex, ethnic group, marital status, occupation or alcohol consumption) is limited. Each variable added to the mix adds more strata to the analysis. The point is reached when finding sufficient subjects to fill the strata becomes prohibitive. To avoid the problem, investigators often base selection of control subjects on characteristics that have been specified in advance. For every case, a control will be chosen who *matches* the

TABLE 8-4

Relative Risk* of Oral Cancer by Level of Smoking and Alcohol Consumption

Alcohol** (ounces/day)	Smoking (Cigarette Equivalents/Day)			
	None	Less than 20	20-39	40 or more
None	1.0	1.5	1.4	2.4
Less than 0.4	1.4	1.7	3.2	3.3
0.4–1.5	1.6	4.4	4.5	8.2
1.6 or more	2.3	4.1	9.6	15.5

*Expressed relative to the baseline risk of 1.0 for those who neither smoke nor drink.
**0.4 ounce equals 1 oz. whiskey or 4 oz. wine or 8 oz. beer.
Source: Based on Rothman & Keller (8).

case with respect to age, sex, ethnic group, and so on. We encountered this concept in Chapter 6, with the study of social factors and tuberculosis in Firland Sanitorium.

Matching requires more effort at the outset to identify appropriate controls but makes analysis of data more efficient. There are many subject characteristics that can be matched— age, sex, race, occupation, social class, and marital status are frequently used—but one needs to be as parsimonious as possible. Each characteristic added to the list makes finding a matching control more difficult.

It also should be recognized that only factors that are likely to confound relationships between exposures and disease should be matched. The goal is to control confounding, so one needn't match for color of eyes or hairstyle, if these are unlikely to relate to either exposure or disease. Nor should factors that may be exposures themselves be matched. These will, by definition, have no differential frequency when cases and controls are compared. If workers with lung cancer were matched by occupation, for example, exposure to asbestos fibers as a risk might go unrecognized. Those who work in ships or other asbestos trades and are exposed to the carcinogen would have been deliberately balanced in the two groups. In this situation, *overmatching* has occurred.

Appropriate selection of cases and controls is not the only challenge to designing case-control studies. The information obtained on risks and exposures from the 2 groups must be of comparable quality. Because data are usually gathered by recollection of past habits or exposures, several sources of unequal *ascertainment* are possible. Human memory is fallible. People forget. A loss of information through faulty recollection usually affects cases and controls equally; there is no bias. But as we have seen with misclassification of polio cases in vaccine trials, these errors dampen differences between case and control groups.

Recollections of the past can be influenced by the present. It is human nature for people with health problems to seek explanations for their plight. What brought on their sickness? Was it something they did? Or didn't do? They search their memories for clues and, sometimes, in an eagerness for answers, distort, unintentionally, the past. An exposure to a medication that might be linked to an adverse reaction may be exaggerated, or a habit that might contribute to illness like smoking or overeating be downplayed. Almost invariably, cases have probed their memories more extensively than have controls. Preferential recall, whether distorted or, more accurately remembered can lead to bias. This *recall bias* can operate in two directions: overstating or underestimating differences between cases and controls.

One can easily imagine recall bias operating in the studies of cigarette smoking and lung cancer. If subjects are convinced that cigarettes are the cause of their disease and that they are victims of the scheming tobacco industry, their recollection of cigarette exposure might prove greater than it actually was. On the other hand, if subjects are chagrined by their past habits, an underestimate of tobacco use might be reported. As it happens, most smoking histories, when they are verified by other means, turn out to be quite accurate.

Those who gather data are susceptible to information bias. If interviewers are aware of the research hypothesis or of associations that are anticipated, cases and controls may be dealt with differently. Cases may be questioned more extensively or prompted for responses. Wynder and Graham worried that because Wynder himself conducted so many of the subject interviews (and was obviously aware of the research questions being addressed) investigator bias could have crept in. He might have worked more diligently to discover smoking among lung cancer cases than among controls. Accordingly, a substudy was conducted in which 2 nonmedical interviewers with no knowledge of the subject's diagnosis or study objectives collected smoking histories. Smoking patterns elicited by this independent pair looked very similar to those Wynder obtained. *Interviewer bias* was not in evidence. Levin and colleagues were fortunate. Because smoking data were gathered from patients on admission, before diagnoses were confirmed or research hypotheses proposed, information bias is minimized. Unfortunately, it is rare that case-control studies find that such useful data have been collected before the research starts.

The biases we have seen may produce associations that are not causal. Selecting cases in which the diagnosis has been influenced by the presence of the factor under scrutiny (toxic shock) or of controls that poorly represent the general population (patients told to stop smoking, drinking coffee, and so on) can create biased associations. An information bias created by differential recall or an interviewer's variable probing can do the same.

It is also possible that associations are simply due to *sampling variation*. This problem is just like the subject allocation issue described in Chapter 6. Returning to the example of a coin tossed 10 times, we know that an equal number of heads and tails is not always the result. We may see 7 heads and 3 tails, 6 tails and 4 heads or even 1 tail and 9 heads. We also understand if we persist with repeated trials of 10 tosses or with increased numbers of tosses, say 100, in every trial, that, on average, we'll get a 50/50 split.

This illustration captures the essence of sampling variation. (It's also known as chance.) In trying to find the true proportion of heads and tails for a tossed coin, we have used samples (of 10) to estimate the true state of affairs. We are really trying to find the proportion of heads and tails among *all* coin tosses—an experiment most would find too tedious to perform. We use samples to produce estimates of this "larger truth" but must accept that samples sometimes miss the mark. We obtain 7 heads and 3 tails instead of 5 and 5 and simply say, "it is the play of chance."

Sampling variation also plays a role in medical studies. Every time a group of lung cancer cases is collected, it is a sample of the larger population of cancer patients. And, as with samples of tossed coins, some variation in the characteristics of these individuals is likely from sample to sample. In trying to find the true smoking frequency for "all" cancer patients we obtain a prevalence of 88% in one sample of cases and 82% in another. This variability relates to sample size. Smaller samples give more variability, larger samples less. Just as with tossed coins, variations of 1 or 2 subjects in a sample size of 10 have a much greater impact than in the sample of 100.

When associations between exposures and disease are being assessed, sampling variability must be considered. Do different smoking frequencies of lung cancer cases and controls represent the true state of affairs, or are they simply caprices of sampling? Statistical procedures are available to help with this question. Calculations can estimate the likelihood that sampling variability explains the differences observed.* The results of these procedures

---

* The specifics of these are beyond our present purposes, but can be found in basic statistics texts.

are summarized as probability statements, or *p values*, that we interpret as "the likelihood that chance could explain the findings." These come in notations such as "$p = .05$" or "$p < .01$" and indicate that the probability of seeing a difference as large or larger than the one observed by chance is only 5 in 100 or less than 1 in 100. The smaller the *p* value, the less likely is an association due to chance. Wynder and Graham and Levin and colleagues applied statistical tests to their work and discovered that the differences in smoking frequencies they found would have occurred from sampling variation less than 1 in 100 times. Chance is an *unlikely* explanation for the association between smoking and lung cancer. An association that survives the challenges of *chance, bias* and *confounding* becomes a strong candidate for a causal relationship.

When the Surgeon General's Report (3) appeared in 1964, just months before Ed Murrow's death, the experts who compiled the document thoroughly reviewed the evidence that linked smoking with lung cancer.* They examined data from animal experiments, from pathology and autopsy work, and from studies on human populations. Among the latter, they discovered 29 published studies similar to those of Wynder and Graham and Levin and colleagues that compared smoking in lung cancer patients with controls. When these studies were scrutinized for bias, confounding, and the role of chance, the association between smoking and lung cancer persisted. But even that was not enough. Before they proclaimed cause, the experts subjected the evidence to a further set of tests.

First, they looked at the *consistency* of the association. Did various studies produce similar findings? Did the results all point in the same direction? Did differing groups of study subjects show like results? The consistency was striking. Every one of the 29 studies found a relationship between cigarette smoking and lung cancer: studies on both men and women, studies that were large and small, studies that came from Europe, Australia, and Japan, as well as the United States. The findings were similar when cases came from the general population, from clinics, or from hospitals, and when controls were chosen from hospitals, clinics, or general groups.

---

* They also dealt with other cancers, respiratory disease, and cardiovascular disease, but lung cancer stood out as the major emphasis of the report.

Regardless of whether studies used data collected from patients themselves or from relatives, employed personal interview or questionnaire, each showed a positive link between cigarettes and lung cancer.

The *strength of the association* was a second test. How substantial were the risks of smoking? Several of the studies gave estimates of the magnitude of risk. As we have noted, Wynder and Graham showed an odds ratio of approximately 13 to 1—a very substantial liability linked to cigarettes. Estimates of risk in other studies were similar, in the neighborhood of 10 to 1—a strong association.

Another feature that helps build the case for cause is the demonstration of a *dose effect*. If risks increase as the degree of exposure rises, the evidence for cause is enhanced. This relationship was also found. Table 8-5 depicts the rise in risk when Wynder and Graham's data are analyzed by comparing cases in each category of smoking intensity with non-smoking controls. Odds ratios rise steadily, from 2.4 among the lightest smokers to almost 30 in the heaviest smoking groups.

The *time relationship* between the associated factors should be plausible. This means sorting eggs from chicks. Exposure must precede disease. Sometimes in case-control studies temporal relationships are not clear. When studying the causes of childhood obesity, for example, researchers find that obese children report less physical activity than do controls. But does a lack of exercise

TABLE 8-5

Odds Ratio for Lung Cancer by Category of Smoking (Compared with Nonsmokers)

Smoking Category	Odds Ratio
Light (1–9 cigarettes/day)	2.4
Moderately heavy (10–15 cigarettes/day)	5.9
Heavy (16–20 cigarettes/day)	10.9
Excessive (21–34 cigarettes/day)	29.6
Chain (35 or more cigarettes/day)	29.7
All smokers	12.8

Source: Based on Wynder & Graham (6).

bring on obesity or are these children less active because they are obese? As smoking begins years before lung cancer is found, this requirement seems satisfied.

Coherence is a final test of an association. Does the evidence from other sources support the epidemiologic findings? Are study results supported by other knowledge from the realms of biology and health? In the cigarette–lung cancer story there are a number of supporting chapters. The ecologic studies we have reviewed that link cigarette consumption and lung cancer over time and across geography are examples of supporting evidence. An explanation of the male-female disparity in cancer rates also helps. Other suggested causes of the lung cancer epidemic—influenza, industrial pollution, and auto exhaust—can't account for this difference, since men and women were equally exposed. Smoking is another matter. Women took up cigarettes later than men. In 1955, a national survey indicated that 65% of men were current smokers compared with only 32% of women; 23% of males had never smoked, compared with more than 67% of females (3, p. 177). The effect of duration is still more evidence. The longer individuals smoke and the younger they take up the habit, the greater is their risk. (It is a variation of the dose effect phenomenon.) Ex-smokers show declining risk. Risk falls as the length of time since stopping grows. Support also comes from the pathology laboratory. Specimens of lungs from smokers who do not have lung cancer commonly show damaged bronchial lining cells. These cells display "precancerous" changes that rise in frequency as the amount of smoking increases. Animals exposed to cigarette smoke also demonstrate cellular changes and tumors. The list goes on.

The rules for claiming cause are not immutable. Often there is room for challenge and debate, but the evidence produced by the Surgeon General's Report was powerful, to say the least. Since 1964, the evidence has grown even more compelling. Dozens of studies on many different populations, using a variety of research techniques, have all reinforced the same message: Cigarette smoking causes lung cancer.

Forty years have passed since Ed Murrow was diagnosed with lung cancer and the Surgeon General's report was issued. The epidemic has gone on. In 1984, 1 in every 1000 American men was diagnosed with lung cancer. That was the peak rate of new cases.

The year 1990 saw the greatest number of lung cancer deaths, with almost 93,000 men succumbing. More recent figures show some respite. As the 21st century begins, just over 90,000 new cases are appearing annually in men, and the rate has dipped slightly to 86 per 100,000. The mortality rate is down 15% from its high a decade earlier. For women, the story differs. As noted, women started smoking later, so their lung cancer epidemic also had a later course. In the 1980s, lung cancer deaths overtook deaths from breast cancer among women. Only now are rates starting to level. Still, the number of new cases in women is approaching that in men; 80,000 annually in the first years of the new century (9).

When Murrow contracted his lung cancer, the outlook wasn't good. Because, as was his case, the disease is usually discovered only after it has become invasive, medical treatment offers scant hope of cure. In Murrow's time, only 7% of lung cancer victims survived 5 years or more. That bleak statistic has improved little. Current 5-year survival figures for men are in the neighborhood of 13%; women fare slightly better, at 17%. This means that the best hope for a solution is prevention. And prevention means attacking the most pervasive cause of the disease—the cigarette.

A variety of solutions to the smoking problem have surfaced since the Surgeon General's Report. Some are personal interventions aimed at helping those who already smoke to stop: nicotine gum and patches, self-help groups, and hypnosis. Broader prevention programs, often mounted at governmental levels, include anti-smoking media campaigns; laws restricting sales to minors; banning smoking in airplanes, restaurants, and other public places; and taxing sales to drive down consumption. Public funding as well as punitive awards from lawsuits against tobacco companies now support statewide programs in tobacco control. At present, smoking patterns vary considerably from state to state. In tobacco-growing Kentucky, for example, 31% of people over the age of 18 smoke; in California the figure is 17%. Per capita consumption in the 2 states ranges from 153 packs of cigarettes per year in Kentucky to only 38 in California. In Kentucky one of those packs carries an average cost of $2.59, where in California a smoker must be prepared to pay a dollar more for every pack.

Still, as a nation, we smoke far less than in Ed Murrow's day. In 1965, when Murrow died, more than 50% of U.S. men and 33%

of women smoked cigarettes. In 2001, there were 46 million smokers, but that number translates to a prevalence of just over 25% in
males and 22% in females (10). In no small part, this healthy shift
is due to countless stories from the print and broadcast media on
the causal link between smoking and lung cancer. These stories
have been based upon a mass of research data that has confirmed
and enlarged upon the hazards of cigarette smoke, hazards not
only to the smoker but to those who breathe his sidestream smoke
or who are born of smoking mothers. It is a mountain of facts that
looms with a single message.

Ed Murrow was among the first in the media to call attention to
the possible connection. But, good newsman that he was, Murrow
was a skeptic. When he broadcast his two *See It Now* programs, he,
himself, was unconvinced of the relationship. Such reservation may
have been denial, given his personal addiction. Or, it may simply
have reflected the kind of intellect for which he was admired, the
critical mind that requires firm evidence. Now, almost 50 years later,
it is hard to think that even Murrow would not be convinced.

REFERENCES

1. Persico JE. *Edward R. Murrow: An American Original.* New
   York: McGraw-Hill; 1988.
2. Kendrick A. *Prime Time: The Life of Edward R. Murrow.*
   Boston: Little, Brown & Co.; 1969.
3. *Smoking and Health: Report of the Advisory Committee to the
   Surgeon General of the Public Health Service.* Public Health
   Service Publication No. 1103. Rockville, MD: U.S.
   Department of Health, Education & Welfare; 1964.
4. *Smoking, Tobacco and Cancer Program: 1985–1989 status
   report.* Bethesda, MD: Department of Health and Human
   Services (NIH publication no. 90-3107); 1990.
5. Doll R. Etiology of lung cancer. *Advances Cancer Res.*
   1955; 3:1–50.
6. Wynder EL, Graham EA. Tobacco smoking as a possible
   etiologic factor in bronchiogenic carcinoma: A study of
   six hundred and eighty-four proved cases. *JAMA.* 1950;
   143:329–336.

7. Levin ML, Goldstein H, Gerhardt PR. Cancer and tobacco smoking: A preliminary report. *JAMA*. 1950; 143:336–338.

8. Rothman K, Keller AZ. The effect of joint exposure to alcohol and tobacco on risk of cancer of the mouth and pharynx. *J Chron Dis*. 1972.

9. Ries LAG, Eisner M, Kosary C. *SEER Cancer Review, 1975–2000*. Bethesda, MD: National Cancer Institute; 2003.

10. Centers for Disease Control and Prevention. Cigarette smoking among adults—United States, 2001. *Morb Mortal Wkly Rep*. 2003; 52(40):953–956.

CHAPTER 9

Searching America's Heart: The Framingham Study

Framingham, Massachusetts, is proud of its 300 years as a community. From the first, the settlement was faithful to its name, derived from Saxon words that mean "house for strangers." It provided refuge for families fleeing the Salem witchcraft frenzy in the 1690s and later would be home to immigrants from Ireland and Italy. The town contributed to the founding of our nation when it raised two companies of minutemen that marched to Concord in April 1775. (Unfortunately, they arrived too late to hear the famous "shot" that changed the world.)

Early 19th-century Framingham's location on the major trade route connecting Boston and New York propelled its growth. As many as 17 coaches daily rumbled down the turnpike through town center, a boon to local liveries, inns, and taverns. In 1835 a rail line was built along its southern edge, which fostered more development. With water power from the nearby Sudbury River available, mills were built, first for corn and lumber, later to make wool and cotton textiles. Factories increased in number through the century, producing carpets, straw hats, shoes, and paper articles.

By the middle of the 20th century the town was thriving. The old turnpike had been replaced with the nation's first paved divided highway. The thoroughfare, known simply as Route 9, was roundly cursed by locals for the traffic snarls it caused. Dennison Manufacturing, the bulwark of town commerce and principal employer since 1897, was so well known for its paper labels that some dubbed Framingham as "Tag Town." A 2.9 million-square-foot General Motors assembly plant had just been built and provided jobs to 4000 townspeople. The facility produced 200,000 vehicles a year and was so large that workers needed bicycles to get from one end of the factory to the other. And the first covered shopping complex east of the Mississippi River, a futuristic apparition known as Shopper's World, was poised to inaugurate its escalators. The complex harbored 44 retail shops and featured the largest unsupported domed building in the country, designed, in keeping with the spirit of the times, to look like a flying saucer that had just touched down.

Framingham was a meat-and-potatoes kind of place. It was not unlike many post–World War II American communities, peopled with small shop owners and plant workers. Many owed their homes and had a Chevrolet or Studebaker car that took them to work or shopping. Little thought was given to exercise beyond that acquired in daily routines. Modern conveniences were making lives easier. New Bendix washers and Sunbeam Mixmasters promised to "save labor" and increase time for fun. Chlorodent toothpaste with chlorophyll made breaths fresher; Toni home permanents made easy curls affordable, and Lustre Crème shampoo turned every woman into a "dream-girl." Released from the rationing of the war, people consumed large quantities of meat and eggs—often twice a day. Cans of Underwood Deviled Ham, Hormel's Spam, and Dinty Moore Beef Stew were prominent on grocer's shelves. Armour's Treet, a blend of pork shoulder and sugar cured ham, was promoted as the perfect dish when served on buttered toast and topped with melted American cheese. Family time was prized. Evenings after supper Dad lit up his Camel cigarette, then everyone collected around the marvelous new television set, to laugh at comic, Milton Berle. Contentment was high.

But with prosperity came liabilities. A chronic disease far more pervasive than the lung cancer we have just explored was showing a dramatic rise. Afflictions of the cardiovascular system—the heart and blood vessels—were growing at an alarming rate. Of particular concern was coronary heart disease, or CHD. Characterized by compromised blow flow to the heart, the most obvious and feared of its manifestations were "heart attacks" and sudden death. In 1900, heart disease caused 27,000 deaths in the United States. It was responsible for 8% of total deaths, with a rate of 40 per 100,000 population. By midcentury, heart disease accounted for 37% of deaths; the rate had risen to 356 per 100,000, and the disease was claiming over half a million lives each year.*

CHD is one member of a group of related conditions known as cardiovascular disease (CVD) that stem from a common pathology. The principle problem carries several names: arteriosclerosis, atherosclerosis, or hardening of the arteries. As the names suggest, the process involves a thickening or hardening of these arteries from buildup of deposits, inside the vessels. Atherosclerosis begins when the inside lining of an artery is injured. This injury may occur from abnormal flow or irritant substances within the blood. Inflammatory cells rush in to repair the damage, but in the process they aggravate the problem. Cellular debris begins to accumulate within the vessel wall as fat deposits. Small mounds, or plaques, are formed, which protrude into the lumen of the artery and impede blood flow. Arteries throughout the body are affected, reducing circulation to vital organs: the limbs, the brain, and most conspicuously, the heart.

In CHD the fundamental difficulty lies with the vessels that bring blood to the heart. These are the coronary arteries that "crown" or circumscribe the organ. As plaque develops over time and supply of oxygen is compromised, characteristic symptoms occur. Predominant of these is chest pain, brought on by exertion and relieved by rest, known as angina pectoris (pain in the chest). An English doctor named William Heberden described the condition so well 230 years ago that his contribution is still found in current medical texts:

> There is a disorder of the breast marked with strong and peculiar symptoms, considerable for the kind of danger belonging to it, and not extremely rare....They who are afflicted with it, are seized while they are walking (more especially if it be up hill, and soon after eating) with a painful and most disagreeable sensation in the breast which seems as if it would extinguish life, if it were to increase or to continue; but the moment they stand still, all this uneasiness vanishes. (1)

---

* Not all heart disease is due to CHD. Other causes such as infections and rheumatic heart disease are included in these figures. In the first years of the century, these accounted for a sizable portion of deaths. By the 1950s, most heart disease deaths were due to CHD.

Angina is a first hallmark of coronary insufficiency brought on by CHD. When disease progresses and an artery becomes entirely blocked, the problem is life threatening. Lacking any blood supply, heart muscle dies. It looses its ability to contract as a pump and to conduct the charged impulses that coordinate contractions. This is a heart attack, a coronary occlusion, or, in the inscrutable terminology of medicine, a *myocardial infarction* (heart muscle death). Heart attacks can be preceded by months of premonitory angina or happen suddenly, with no prior warning. Usually they are accompanied by immobilizing, crushing chest pain, but sometimes they are "silent." Sudden death can be the only notice that CHD is present.

In 1948, the cause of CHD was not known, though theories were about. Many thought it might be *multicausal*, that a variety of factors—characteristics of a person and the environment—interacted to produce disease. Included on the suspect list were high blood pressure, obesity, fat in the diet, cigarette smoking, and economic status. But there was little evidence supporting any of these claims for cause. Research was sparse. Even adequate descriptive studies, detailing the *who, when, and where* of CHD were minimal. It seemed that men were more often affected than women, that likelihood of illness advanced with age, and that all regions of the country were experiencing the epidemic. But little more was clear. If any efforts were to be mounted to reverse the trends, more information was desperately required.

Physicians in the U.S. Public Health Service recognized the problem. They also realized that its solution would necessitate a new approach. The traditional research tack, of identifying cases of disease after they had occurred and describing them, seemed unlikely to produce results. The disease developed so insidiously, and had so many antecedent candidates for cause, that untangling histories of past habits and exposures seemed untenable. What they proposed instead broke new ground. Rather than starting with subjects who were already ill, as had been done successfully with lung cancer, they would begin with subjects who were well. These subjects would be examined thoroughly and their habits recorded. Then periodically, they would be reassessed, and, over time, those who developed disease would be discovered. A clear relationship between the factors that precede disease and CHD would be established.

It was a clever plan, to track a group of subjects forward in time and watch for disease. The design was dubbed a *cohort*, or a *follow-up study*, after the concept of assembling a group and the forward action of the study. It was also a plan of unparalleled ambition. How many well individuals would need to be followed to obtain sufficient numbers who develop heart disease? How many years would be required for this to happen? It was new territory. The study would have to be much larger and last much longer than any research endeavor previously attempted. But the problem they were facing was enormous and scientists at the Public Health Service's National Institutes of Health believed that the reward would justify the effort.

It was decided that the project was most likely to succeed if efforts concentrated on a single community rather than attempting a cross-section of the country that would necessitate the management of many sites. They reckoned that a sample of about 6000 people would produce sufficient cases of CHD for reasonable analysis. These should be between the ages of 30 and 60; younger subjects would be less likely to develop heart disease, and older ones might already be too far along the road. The study would run for 20 years. A huge commitment would be needed, from the government who would fund the study; from the research team that would organize and implement the plan, and from any community that would volunteer to provide the subjects.

Typically American, Framingham was just the place. Among its population of 28,000 were enough people in the 30- to 60-year age bracket (about 10,000) to find sufficient subjects. Still, the town was small enough that folks knew one another; communication was easy. The town-meeting style of governance meant that citizens were accustomed to group participation. Thirty years before, the town had agreed to be a testing ground for a large demonstration project on TB control. With assistance from the Massachusetts State Health Department and state medical society, and with local doctors in support, the town was approached, and citizens agreed to take part. An executive committee of residents was formed to help with logistics and recruitment, and the Framingham Heart Study was underway (2).

As there were more available adults of the appropriate age than were required, a random sample of the target population was identified. Then each of these potential subjects was asked by a fellow citizen recruiter to participate. Agreeing meant an interview that probed for all sorts of medical history and habits and a physical exam of greater thoroughness than most had ever had. Then there were chest x-rays, an electrocardiogram, and a multiplicity of blood tests. The process was to be repeated every 2 years. Any problems uncovered would be referred to the subject's own doctor. Study organizers asked 6510 individuals to join. Of this number, 4469—2024 men and 2445 women—agreed and were examined. Then the clock began and everyone sat back to wait.

Four years and 2 biennial examinations later the investigators took their first peek at the results (2). Of the 4469 that were initially enrolled, 76 were found to have CHD at the first examination. That meant they already had angina or evidence (from their cardiogram) of a previous heart attack or coronary artery disease. This is *prevalence*, the amount of existing CHD in the population at a specific point in time. It was twice as high in men (24 per 1000 versus 11 per 1000) and 2-fold greater in the older ages.

Prevalence gives a useful estimate of the burden of disease at a moment in time. Studies that yield prevalence are also known as *cross-sectional*, for the "slice-in-time" data they produce. They are often helpful in establishing a baseline look at health conditions preparatory to more detailed follow-up efforts, or they can be useful by themselves to map trends in diseases or exposures and risk factors over time (see Figure 9-1). Cross-sectional studies are usually efficient and can be accomplished relatively rapidly. However, time relationships can get confused. Since data are collected all at once, it isn't always clear whether exposures or diseases happen first. If a subject is found to have CHD and is obese, did obesity bring on heart disease, or did angina (heart disease) prompt inactivity and subsequent weight gain? Nor does the prevalence approach capture all the cases of disease. Sudden deaths due to heart attack, which were an important outcome of the Framingham study, are missed, for example. The longer a disease condition lingers, the more likely it will be included in a cross-sectional survey.

The more intriguing data lay ahead, in the events occurring in the 4 years that had passed since enrollment. Of those who did not have CHD initially (4469, less the 76 with existing disease), how

FIGURE 9-1

Detecting Coronary Heart Disease Risk Factors:
An Exhibition

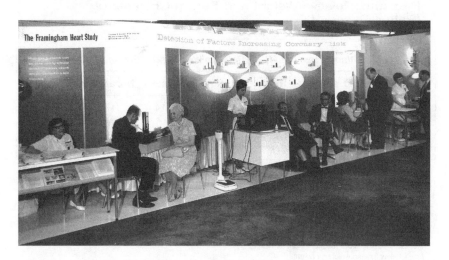

Source: Courtesy Framingham Heart Study.

many experienced onset of angina, heart attack, or sudden cardiac death? This was the essence of the cohort approach: new cases. These yield the *incidence* of disease, the number of new cases in a population over a specified period of time. Unlike prevalence, incidence is a rate; it includes time as a dimension—new cases per 1000 population during a month or over a year. Incidence can capture sudden deaths and, since cohorts are tracked over time, sort out time relationships for risk factors and disease outcomes.

The 4-year incidence of CHD was 22 per 1000. Ninety-seven subjects—65 men and 32 women—experienced heart attacks, died suddenly, or contracted angina (2). Most of them (87%) were above the age of 45. The recognized relationships of age and sex to CHD were substantiated. Incidence was higher among men and increased with age. Things got more interesting when investigators began to probe other predictors of disease. Three potential risk factors received particular scrutiny: blood pressure (hypertension), weight (overweight/obesity), and serum cholesterol (elevated). Table 9-1 displays the findings for males, ages 45 to 62 (the group with most

TABLE 9-1

Incidence of Coronary Heart Disease (CHD) During Four Year Follow-up for 898 Males* Ages 45-62 by Blood Pressure, Relative Weight and Serum Cholesterol (Rate = Cases/1000)

Category	Blood Pressure (1)		Relative Weight (2)		Serum Cholesterol (3)	
	No. at Risk	Rate	No. at Risk	Rate	No. at Risk	Rate
High	206	87	176	114	172	122
Medium	335	66	320	50	265	45
Low	310	26	397	40	445	40

*Numbers at risk may not add to total because of missing values
(1) Blood pressure:
    High = definite hypertension or hypertensive heart disease
    Medium = borderline hypertension or possible hypertensive heart disease
    Low = normotension
(2) Relative weight:
    High = 13% or more above median weight for height
    Medium = 0–12% above median weight for height
    Low = below median weight for height
(3) Serum cholesterol:
    High = 260 milligrams percent and above
    Medium = 225–259 milligrams percent
    Low = less than 225 milligrams percent
Source: Based on Dawber (2).

new CHD). Each of the 3 characteristics is associated with heart disease. Those with highest blood pressure have the higher rates of CHD than those with the lowest levels. The same is true for weight and cholesterol.

To quantify these relationships, a ratio can be constructed that compares the rates (cases per 1000) for the highest and lowest groups. For blood pressure, the ratio is 87/1000 over 26/1000, or 3.3. The comparable ratios for weight and cholesterol are 2.8 (114/1000 over 40/1000) and 3.0 (122/1000 over 40/1000), respectively. These are *rate* or *risk ratios*. They convey a message akin to the odds ratios discussed in Chapter 8. Risk ratios express the increased (or decreased) likelihood of disease conferred by an exposure or characteristic. They differ slightly from odds ratios. Risk ratios tell us the relative chance of developing heart disease if hypertension or high cholesterol is present; odds ratios offer the less straightforward message of the likelihood of having smoked for those who have lung cancer. Both ratios are used as expressions of *relative risk*. Risk ratios are generally preferred but can be obtained only from cohort (not case-control) studies.

A risk ratio or relative risk higher than 1 indicates a greater likelihood of disease when the factor is present; a ratio less than 1 that disease is less likely. Relative risks are translated into prose in several ways. An exposure with a relative risk of 3.0 "triples the chance of disease," or "increases disease 300%," or "causes 3 times the risk." All three expressions report the same finding. The magnitude of relative risks found in health studies varies considerably. The 2- to 3-fold risks for CHD are meaningful multiples. The 10-fold risk seen with smoking and lung cancer is considered high and is not commonly encountered. Workers exposed to asbestos fiber while installing insulation in buildings or ships have a risk of lung cancer that is 60 times higher than that of the general population, but ratios of such magnitude are rare. Most relative risks are much lower, often less than 2.0. These can still be important. A number of studies find that women taking postmenopausal estrogens have a relative risk for breast cancer of 1.3 to 1.4.

The risk ratios derived from Table 9-1 implicated all 3 factors: blood pressure, excess weight, and cholesterol. But high blood pressure has long been known to be strongly associated with overweight. Obese people generally have higher blood pressures. The question arises whether both factors play a role in CHD. Or is only one factor responsible and the second simply traveling as a marker? Is confounding taking place? The data in Table 9-2 address this concern. Here, rates of CHD are displayed in strata—high, medium, and low for each of the three characteristics, while the other risk factors are held constant at medium or low levels. A gradient of risk is seen for each: from a rate of 100 cases per 1000 for blood pressure to only 17 per 1000; from 57 per 1000 to 28 per thousand for weight; from 80 per thousand to 13 per thousand for cholesterol. This means that blood pressure, weight, and cholesterol each independently influences risk for CHD. Confounding is not the explanation.

If each factor by itself plays a role in heart disease, what happens if a subject has more than one factor? Table 9-3 on page 219 shows rates of CHD when varying combinations of risk factors are present. Subjects with 2 or 3 high factors are clearly at the greatest risk, with 143 cases for every 1000 participants. Those in the low

TABLE 9-2

Incidence of Coronary Heart Disease (CHD) During Four
Year Follow-up for 877 Males* Ages 45-62 by Blood
Pressure, Relative Weight and Serum Cholesterol, Partially
Controlled for Other Variables (Rate = Cases/1000)

Blood Pressure (1)	Relative Weight (2)	Serum Cholesterol (3)	No. at Risk	Rate
High	Medium or low	Medium or low	91	100
Medium	Medium or low	Medium or low	242	37
Low	Medium or low	Medium or low	240	17
Medium or low	**High**	Medium or low	87	57
Medium or low	**Medium**	Medium or low	198	25
Medium or low	**Low**	Medium or low	284	28
Medium or low	Medium or low	**High**	112	80
Medium or low	Medium or low	**Medium**	178	51
Medium or low	Medium or low	**Low**	304	13

*Numbers at risk may not add to total because of missing values
(1) Blood pressure:
   High = definite hypertension or hypertensive heart disease
   Medium = borderline hypertension or possible hypertensive heart disease
   Low = normotension
(2) Relative weight
   High = 13% or more above median weight for height
   Medium = 0–12% above median weight for height
   Low = below median weight for height
(3) Serum cholesterol
   High = 260 milligrams percent and above
   Medium = 225–259 milligrams percent
   Low = less than 225 milligrams percent
Source: Based on Dawber (2).

category for all 3 have the lowest rate: only 10 per 1000. Having multiple factors adds to the risk. The risk ratio for those with 2 or more
high ratings compared with those who are low for all 3 is 14.3.

Other insights were revealed as the findings from this landmark study were unfurled. Some reflected on the methodology. The
value of the study's design lay in its prospective approach, in the
capacity to assess risk factors before disease was manifest. There was
also virtue in the view it offered on the state of the community's
health: a snapshot of the health of hearts in a typical New England
town. The use of *random sampling* meant that subjects selected should
present a representative picture of the town. Every adult in the

TABLE 9-3

Incidence of Coronary Heart Disease (CHD) During Four Year Follow-up for 877 Males* Ages 45-62 by Various Combinations of Blood Pressure (1), Relative Weight (2) and Serum Cholesterol (3) (Rate = Cases/1000)

	No. at Risk	Rate	Risk Ratio**
High on two or more	105	143	14.3
High on one only	290	79	7.9
Medium on two or more	186	38	3.8
Medium on one only	198	25	2.5
All low	98	10	1.0

*Numbers at risk may not add to total because of missing values
**Ratio of rate compared to "all low"
(1) Blood pressure
   High = definite hypertension or hypertensive heart disease
   Medium = borderline hypertension or possible hypertensive heart disease
   Low = normotension
(2) Relative weight
   High = 13% or more above median weight for height
   Medium = 0–12% above median weight for height
   Low = below median weight for height
(3) Serum cholesterol
   High = 260 milligrams percent and above
   Medium = 225–259 milligrams percent
   Low = less than 225 milligrams percent
Source: Based on Dawber (2).

eligible age range had an equal chance of being included—at least in theory. Unfortunately, some of the best laid plans don't always work (3). Not all of those selected by the random method chose to participate. Table 9-4 shows this.

Of the more than 6500 people selected only 2 in 3 were examined and became part of the cohort. Over 2000 of those eligible did not participate. Some moved away from Framingham, some died, and some were too ill or incapacitated to join; 1464 "refused." Could such nonparticipation have implications? Could nonparticipants be less well as well as less cooperative? If those who don't take part have risk profiles or outcomes that differ from those who do, bias can occur. There is evidence such was the case. The demographics of participants and nonparticipants differed in a number of ways. For one, 75% of women below the age of 45 participated; the same was true for only 66% of men. For older men and women (the group most at risk), the figure fell

TABLE 9-4

Age-Adjusted Death Rates for Framingham Subjects by
Level of Participation and Reason for Nonparticipation

	Number	% of eligible	Age-Adjusted Death Rate (per 1000)	
			Men	Women
Total eligible	6532	100	8.9	4.3
Examined/participated	4494	68.8	8.2	3.2
Not examined	2038	31.2	10.4	6.9
Moved from area	426	6.5	4.6	3.6
Died	74	1.1	—	—
Ill or incapacitated	74	1.1	14.8	11.9
Refused	1464	22.4	11.9	7.3

Source: Based on Gordon (3).

to 60%. Response rates also varied by sections of the town, from 57 to 76%, depending on the precinct—a possible marker of differences in socioeconomic status. But most revealing were the links between participation and subsequent mortality obtained from death certificate data (shown on the right-hand side of Table 9-4).

Death rates, adjusted for age, are twice as high for men as women overall: 8.9 versus 4.3 per 1000. As a group, nonparticipants have higher rates than participants: 27% higher for men and twofold (200%) higher for women. Particularly informative are the subcategories of nonparticipation. Of no surprise is the fact that those ill or incapacitated have the highest rates of death; those who are mobile and move from town have lower rates than typical participants. The figures for those "refusing" are the second highest: 11.9 per 1000 for men and 7.3 per 1000 for women. Clearly nonparticipants are not a random subset of the community. They offer an example of the *selection bias* we encountered back in Chapter 2. Like the people who get flu vaccine or take hormone replacement therapy, their health is not typical of the community at large. This means that data on the prevalence and incidence of CHD in Framingham are likely to underestimate the true picture.

A similar concern arises when subjects are followed over time. Not everyone who joins stays in the study. Some die, some move away, some simply don't return for follow-up examinations. If those who "drop out" or are lost to follow-up differ systematically from the "followed" group, bias can, again, result. Framingham investigators worked hard to keep subjects in the study. But over the years the research ran, it was inevitable that losses would occur. When the measures collected initially on "lost" subjects were reviewed, this group, indeed, showed differences from their continuing counterparts. Blood pressures, weights, and cholesterol levels were all higher on earlier examinations (3).

A few years after the Framingham Heart Study was launched, two distinguished English researchers initiated another cohort study. In October 1951, Richard Doll and A. B. Hill (4) sent out a simple questionnaire to 50,000 men who were registered as doctors in Great Britain. Their survey wasn't lengthy, in hopes that brevity would be the "soul" of good response. It asked for details on the doctors' current smoking habits: when begun, how long continued, type of tobacco used, and so on. The object was to classify this cohort by their smoking exposure and follow their mortality in years to come. Some 34,000 replies were received—a slightly better than two-thirds response. From the outset Doll and Hill recognized that those who chose to answer might not represent the total group. To see if selection bias could be at play, they drew 2 small samples from among those who originally had responded and those who had not. Again, they sent requests for details on smoking habits. His time the previous "nonanswerers" did better: 84% responded. And 28% admitted being moderate or heavy cigarette smokers; only 6% were nonsmokers. In contrast, the comparable figures for those who had previously "answered' were 15 and 21%. Responders had healthier habits. These differences were reflected in the cohort's mortality experience, which was consistently below the death rate for the total population of British doctors.

Selective forces that influence subject entry and follow-up in cohort studies can distort our view of prevalence and incidence. The findings from Framingham and the study of British doctors most likely underestimate true rates of illness in the entire town or physician registry. But risk information gathered from comparisons within the cohorts is less hampered by selection. These findings should have general applicability to groups beyond the confines of the study.

The study of British doctors offered further fuel to the tobacco "fire." Results confirmed the case-control connections between cigarettes and lung cancer. But the study also found that cigarettes contribute to a host of other ills. Mortality rates (the only outcome that was recorded) were higher among smokers for a number of diseases: other cancers such as of the larynx, esophagus, and bladder; other respiratory illness such as emphysema and bronchitis; and coronary heart disease.

The British survey highlights another problem that burdens cohort studies. What happens when subjects alter their risk while the study is in progress? Habits of participants that are found at entry may not persist. The overweight may shed pounds, those with high cholesterol may lower fat intake, hypertensives may seek treatment, and smokers may quit. Those who change become misclassified and, as we have seen before, will tend to obscure differences between exposed and unexposed. In the British study, doctors did change their smoking habits. After 7 years, the researchers resurveyed subjects about current smoking. Some who were initially nonsmokers had begun to smoke. But most shifts were in the opposite direction, men who were smokers when the study began cut down or quit. There were, in fact, 3 subjects who reduced for every 1 who increased the habit (4). Such an imbalance distorts results if subjects remain misclassified according to original categories. If smoking leads to CHD, then those who quit may be at lower risk. They would have fewer adverse outcomes and contribute to an underestimate of smoking risk if they are counted in the smoking group. On the other hand, those who quit may be induced to do so *because* of illness. Symptoms such as angina or bronchitis may prompt cessation. Should these folks be reclassified as nonsmokers, disease would appear more common in the group than would be appropriate.

Risks must be reassessed from time to time. One virtue of the Framingham study was the scheduled reexamination that took place every 2 years. Subjects could be rechecked for blood pressure, weight, and cholesterol, as well as personal habits and resorted to appropriate bins. But how do we treat subjects who change? Do they count as smokers or nonsmokers? Or should there be a category for ex-smokers, since quitting might or might not alter risk? Excluding subjects who change their status means losing hard-earned data. So, shifts in risks need to be accommodated. Subjects can be considered smokers for the intervals they smoke. Someone who smokes for 4 years of a 10-year follow-up and then quits can be counted proportionately in 2 groups. He contributes 4 years as a smoker and 6 years as an ex-smoker. Each subject then produces 10 years of experience, or 10 *person-years*. Many subjects will have consistent risks for all 10 years: 10 person-years of normal blood pressure or high cholesterol. Others will produce a mixture. The use of person-years of cumulative risk helps cohort studies make the most of inevitable change. It also aids when subjects drop out or die before the study has run its full course. Their data can contribute for the time that they participate.

The findings of the study of British doctors added a dimension to the risk discussion (5). Valuable information could be obtained not only from comparing risk ratios but also by looking at *risk difference*. Examining the differences in rates of mortality between those with and without a risk factor or exposure highlights the factor's role in producing a disease within a population. Also called *attributable risk*, risk difference describes the amount of illness that can be blamed on the risk factor. Table 9-5 compares both risk ratios and risk differences for CHD and lung cancer derived from death rates of the British doctors.

TABLE 9-5

Comparative Risks for Lung Cancer and Coronary Heart Disease (CHD) Among Male British Doctors Who Are Smokers and Nonsmokers

Cause of Death	Annual Deaths per 100,000*		Risk Ratio	Risk Difference (per 100,000)	Proportionate Risk Ratio (%)
	Smokers	Nonsmokers			
Lung cancer	140	10	14	130	93
CHD	669	413	1.6	256	38

*Age-adjusted.
Source: Based on Doll & Peto (5).

The table confirms that annual rates of lung cancer death for smokers are much higher than for nonsmokers (140 per 100,000 versus 10 per 100,000). The risk ratio is 14 to 1. These same figures also provide a risk difference of 130 per 100,000. The difference can be thought of as the amount of risk contributed by smoking to smokers' death rates. Attributable risk (risk difference) takes into account the fact that not all blame for lung cancer can be placed on smoking. Other risk factors (industrial exposures, air pollution, radiation, genetic predisposition) contribute as well. However, the proportionate risk contributed by smoking to lung cancer (calculated as the attributable risk of 130/100,000 over the total risk in smokers of 140/100,000) is 93 percent—certainly the lion's share.

For CHD the pattern differs. Death rates for smokers and non-smokers are 669 and 413 per 100,000, respectively. The risk ratio for smoking and CHD is surprisingly low: only 1.6 (669/100,000 over 413/100,000). Smoking appears to play a lesser role in causing CHD than in lung cancer. But there is more to tell. The risk difference indicates that 256 per 100,000 of the CHD deaths among smokers can be attributed to smoking. That's almost twice the rate as that for lung cancer. So, although smoking carries a much higher relative risk for lung cancer, more lives are lost each year to the CHD it produces.

From the public health perspective, this is worthy news. Lung cancer is commonly considered the most important target of efforts to reduce smoking. Yet, despite the less alarming relative risk, and lower proportionate contribution to total CHD mortality (38% of CHD deaths in smokers are due to smoking: $256/100,000 \div 669/100,000 = .38$), more lives might be saved from CHD averted when smoking is reduced. The apparent "role reversal" is simply because the outcomes vary in their frequency. Deaths from CHD are almost 5 times more common than deaths from lung cancer among smokers. So differences in rates between smokers and nonsmokers yield more CHD deaths than do differences for lung cancer, despite the latter's larger relative risk.

There's another element to consider in evaluating risk as well. Not only do some exposures lead to more than one disease (smoking to heart disease, cancers, and bronchitis), but a particular disease may be precipitated by more than one exposure. This is an important lesson of the Framingham Heart Study. Initial concerns focused on CHD. But as the study proceeded, disease outcomes of interest broadened to include such related cardiovascular problems as stroke and heart failure. Heart failure occurs when the muscle pump is weakened and can no longer provide an adequate supply of blood to meet the need of body organs. This can be brought about by high blood pressure, when years of trying to push against constricted arteries exact a toll, or following a heart attack, when damage to parts of the muscle weakens the heart.

When Framingham researchers looked at the role of these two risk factors, they obtained the data shown in Table 9-6 (6). Risk ratios were much larger (worse) for both men and women who had heart attacks. Both were 6 times more likely to develop heart failure than those without heart attacks. Relative risks for hypertension were also elevated (greater than 1), although not as high as heart failure: 2.1 and 3.4 for men and women, respectively. It is evident that heart attack creates a greater risk of heart failure than does high blood pressure.

But differing frequencies again are important. The second column in Table 9-6 shows the prevalence of the 2 risk factors among study subjects. High blood pressure is considerably more common than heart attack. In fact, 60% of both men and women have hypertension, but only 10% of men and 3% of women have suffered heart attacks. This means that, even though relative risk is higher for heart attack, high blood pressure causes more heart failure in the

TABLE 9-6

Comparative Risks for Heart Failure Among Framingham Participants with Hypertension and Heart Attack

Risk Factor	Relative Risk*		Prevalence (%)		Population Attributable Risk (%)	
	Men	Women	Men	Women	Men	Women
Hypertension	2.1	3.4	60	62	39	59
Prior heart attack	6.3	6.0	10	3	34	13

*Adjusted for age and other risk factors
Source: Based on Levy et al. (6).

community, as the right-hand columns of Table 9-6 show. Hypertension contributes to 39% of the cases in men and 59% of the cases in women, compared with the 34% and 13% respective roles for heart attack. This is the *population attributable risk percent* and is another way of using risk difference. Subtracting the rate of heart failure for those *without* exposure (hypertension or heart attack) from the overall rate in the community (including those *with* exposure) and dividing by the overall rate creates the number. The result accounts not only for differences in rates of disease for those with and without a factor but the frequency with which the risk is present. The message is an obvious but important one: When diseases are more common or exposures more prevalent, their importance in a population rises.

Differing types of risk statements can cause confusion. Ratios, as proportions representing increase or decrease, are probably the most familiar. For example: The costs of college education have doubled in the last 10 years. Property taxes have risen 40% since we bought this house. The population of the town has fallen by 12% in just 2 years. But relative risk statements lack important information. They don't reveal the numerators and denominators that were used in their construction. A doubling of tuition or 40% increase in taxes sound dramatic. But their significance depends upon the magnitude of the amounts on which the ratios are based. A tax rise of 40% could mean an extra $400 if the past bill is $1000 or $2400 more if the starting point is $6000. Information on the *differences* between the old and new amounts is likely to be more salient to the beleaguered taxpayer than *ratios*.

A health study that explores potential risks and benefits of hormone replacement therapy (HRT) for postmenopausal women illustrates the complexities inherent in interpreting risk. The Women's Health Initiative (WHI) (7) is a randomized clinical trial created to determine whether replacing estrogen is, on balance, beneficial. Recall from Chapter 2 that a number of observational studies, including well-executed cohort efforts, had suggested HRT improved mortality from CHD. In addition to relieving postmenopausal symptoms, lower risks of osteoporotic fracture and colon cancer had also been found. On the negative side, women taking HRT were more likely to develop breast cancer and, if taking estrogen alone, cancer of the endometrium. There is evidence that hormone users are a selected group (they smoke less, among other factors) and worry that apparent benefits might be artifacts of better underlying health and not the treatment (confounding). With that in mind, the experiment was designed in hopes of clarifying the matter.

From 1993 through 1998, the WHI enrolled more than 16,000 postmenopausal women between the ages of 50 and 79 with intact uteruses from across the United States. These were randomly assigned to receive either an estrogen + progestin combination (the progestin is added to reduce the risk of endometrial cancer) or placebo daily. Investigators estimated that in 8 years time they would have sufficient evidence to show once and for all any advantages of HRT. Best guesses were that hormone therapy would reduce the risk of CHD by 40 to 50%.

The results were a surprise. The trial was stopped early, after only 5.2 years of follow-up. Such cessation is not unheard of. In most medical experiments in which treatments are being compared for serious diseases, agreement is reached before enrollment begins that the trial will be concluded before its full course if results appear convincing that one therapy is superior. This early stopping is to avoid continuing to expose subjects to a treatment that is known to be less effective. But the reverse is also true. Trials can be concluded if excessive risk is found. This was the case in the WHI. Breast cancer occurred more frequently in women taking HRT; so did strokes and pulmonary embolism (blood clots to the lung); and so did CHD. Hip fractures and colorectal cancer were less frequent. The findings are shown in Table 9-7.

Results are presented for 6 major outcomes: CHD, stroke, pulmonary embolism (PE), breast cancer, colorectal cancer, and hip fracture. In addition, there is an overall, global index that combines these 6 principle events and endometrial cancer with deaths from all other causes. In relative terms, risks for CHD are increased almost 30% and 26% for breast cancer; risks for the adverse outcomes of stroke and PE are 41% and 113% greater for estrogen plus progestin (E+P) users. The protective effects seen for hip fracture and colorectal cancer are relative reductions of 34% and 37%, respectively. The global index shows a net increase of *adverse* events of 15%.

This is unhappy news. For many women and their doctors, interpreting these data to make decisions about using HRT is challenging. Heightening one's chances of CHD by 30% or of breast cancer by

TABLE 9-7

Risk of Clinical Outcomes for Women Taking Estrogen Plus Progestin (E + P) or Placebo for an Average of 5.2 Years in the Women's Health Initiative

Outcome	No. of Subjects E + P Years, $n = 8506$	Placebo $n = 8102$	Risk Ratio	% Change	Risk Difference per 10,000 per Year	Risk Difference per 10,000 in 5.2 Years
Coronary heart disease	164	122	1.29	29	7	42
Stroke	127	85	1.41	41	8	44
Pulmonary embolism	70	31	2.13	113	8	44
Breast cancer	166	124	1.26	26	8	42
Colorectal cancer	45	67	0.63	−37	−6	−30
Hip fracture	44	62	0.66	−34	−5	−25
Global index*	751	623	1.15	15	19	114

*Global index = any of 6 events listed or endometrial cancer or any death due to other causes.

Source: Based on Rossouw et al. (7).

26% is a sobering proposition. Again, however, risk ratios tell only part of the story. Missing is a grounding in the absolute magnitude of risk of the adverse outcomes and the risk difference that is associated with HRT. In the 5 years of the study, 751 of the 8506 women taking E + P and 623 of the 8102 placebo takers experienced adverse "global index" outcomes. The risk of one of these adverse events that can be attributed to taking E +P (risk difference) is 114 for every 10,000 who took E +P for 5 years (about 1%). Viewed from an annual perspective, 7 additional women will develop CHD and 8 will develop breast cancer each year for every 10,000 taking E +P.

Risk differences better inform personal decisions because they include denominators, the numbers of women who are *at risk* (take E +P) as well as the numbers who experience increased (or decreased) outcome events. Risk differences also help estimate the larger, public health impact of widespread use of HRT. When events per 10,000 are multiplied by the national figures of those taking the product, the extent of the adverse consequences becomes substantial. Based on estimates of recent use (8), over 6000 "global events" would occur each year among E +P users. Certainly, on the basis of the data from the WHI, thoughts of deploying HRT as a public health strategy for lowering CHD among postmenopausal women have lost appeal. On the other hand, for an individual, whose quality of life is substantially diminished from postmenopausal symptoms, the incremental risks of therapy might be worth taking.

By 1971, the Framingham Heart Study had met its projected goal; 20 years of follow-up had been completed. Tens of thousands of biennial examinations had been performed, and only 5% of the initial participants were unaccounted for. One hundred scientific papers had been published on its findings. The study had become a standard for its type and had provided major keys to unlocking the complex risks of coronary heart disease. But enthusiasm for the project was still high, among the sponsors, the investigators, and the community. It was decided to continue. A new cohort was initiated; 5135 new subjects, 2489 males and 2646 females were launched on a new round of examinations. They were the sons and daughters of the original volunteers.

This "offspring cohort" has now been watched for more than 30 years and helped expand our knowledge, not simply on the risks of CHD, but on conditions such as hearing loss, osteoporosis, cataracts, and dementia. The range of risks identified has also expanded. Infectious agents such as chlamydia, cytomegalovirus, and helicobacter have become subjects of investigation as has the amino acid homocysteine. Cholesterol has been subclassified into a host of distinct lipid proteins that each contributes different degree of risk. Blood samples are now obtained for DNA analysis in hopes that the genetic underpinnings of heart disease will be revealed. The technologies available to track disease have improved. Tools of far greater sophistication than those employed in 1950, now send beams of ultrasound to delineate the structures of the heart and create computerized tomograms to trace the coronary arteries and calculate the density of thinning bones. In 2000, a third generation, a cohort of grandchildren, began.

The risks and health of residents has changed some in the interval. The prevalence of high blood pressure has fallen dramatically since the 1950s. Where 18% of men and 28% of women had substantial elevations, recent data show figures down to 9 and 8%, respectively (9). The shift reflects a marked increase in use of drugs for antihypertensive care: an 11-fold rise for men and 5-fold rise for women. The trends for cigarette smoking have been mixed. Comparisons of 50- to 59-year-old men and women from the original and the offspring cohorts indicate that men have dropped their prevalence by half. Data for women are less encouraging. Prevalence is higher among offspring than their mothers and above the levels of their male contemporaries (31 versus 26%) (10). Cholesterol levels show evidence of some decline. Fewer female offspring are obese but prevalence rose in offspring men.

Overall the news is positive. When comparisons of health were made, the offspring cohort came out well ahead (11). Among those evaluated between ages 55 and 70, fewer men and women in the offspring group perceived themselves in "fair or poor health." They also reported fewer disabilities. Lower frequencies of 4 of the 5 major chronic diseases were found. Only diabetes had increased. The prevalence of cardiovascular disease, hypertension, chronic obstructive pulmonary disease, and arthritis was less among the offspring group.

The town of Framingham has also done well, though not without some bumps along the way. The population is now 67,000, and it is more diverse. Latinos, Asians, and African Americans have joined the sons and daughters of early Irish and Italian immigrants and make up 20% of the population. The economy has been a mixed story. The first 20 years of the heart study saw great growth. From 1950 to 1970, the population jumped from 28,000 to 64,000, almost its present size. Business then was ebullient, with 70 manufacturing establishments, 85 wholesale firms, and 338 retail businesses. Retail sales soared, from 28 million in 1951, when Shopper's World opened, to more than $500 million (12).

But the growth reached a plateau and the recession of the early 1990s was not kind to Framingham. In 1991, the General Motors plant closed and the 4000 jobs were lost. In the wake of that calamity, total employment fell. Jobs dropped by 27% from levels of the mid-1980s. Things have improved since then. New hi-tech businesses have come in; Shopper's World has been redone. The economy has returned to close to prerecession levels, though the type of work in Framingham has changed. Most manufacturing is gone and service industries prevail. Medical, technology, and educational activities are now the mainstays of the town. Community pride and contentment continue to be in evidence, though people still complain about the traffic on Route 9.

REFERENCES

1. Heberden W. Commentaries on the history and cure of diseases. In: Willius FA, Keys, T.E., ed. *Classics in Cardiology, volume I*, NY: Dover Publications; 1961.
2. Dawber TR, Moore FE, Mann GV. Coronary heart disease in the Framingham study. *Am J Public Health*. Apr 1957; 47:4-24.
3. Gordon T, Moore F, Shurtleff D, Dawber T. Some methodologic problems in the long-term study of cardiovascular disease: observations on the Framingham Study. *J Chron Dis*. 1959; 10:186–206.
4. Doll R, Hill AB. Mortality in relation to smoking: ten years' observations of British doctors. *British Medical Journal*. 1964; 1:1399–1410.
5. Doll R, Peto R. Mortality in relation to smoking; 20 years' observations on male British doctors. *British Medical Journal*. 1976; 2:1525–1536.
6. Levy D, Larson MG, Vasan RS, Kannel WB, Ho KK. The progression from hypertension to congestive heart failure. *JAMA*. 1996; 275:1557–1562.
7. Rossouw JE, Anderson GL, Prentice RL, et al. Risks and benefits of estrogen plus progestin in healthy postmenopausal women: principal results from the Women's Health Initiative randomized controlled trial. *JAMA*. 2002; 288:321–333.
8. Keating NL, Cleary PD, Rossi AS, Zaslavsky AM, Ayanian JZ. Use of hormone replacement therapy by postmenopausal women in the United States. *Ann Internal Med*. 1999; 130:545–553.
9. Mosterd A, D'Agostino RB, Silbershatz H, et al. Trends in the prevalence of hypertension, antihypertensive therapy, and left ventricular hypertrophy from 1950 to 1989. *N Engl J Med*. 1999; 340(16):1221–1227.

10. Sytkowski PA, D'Agostino RB, Belanger A, Kannel WB. Sex and time trends in cardiovascular disease incidence and mortality: the Framingham Heart Study, 1950–1989. *Am J Epidemiol.* 1996; 143(4):338–350.

11. Allaire SH, LaValley MP, Evans SR, et al. Evidence for decline in disability and improved health among persons aged 55 to 70 years: the Framingham Heart Study. *Am J Public Health.* 1999; 89(11):1678–1683.

12. Sanders I, Gelfand D. *Framingham: A Profile of a Rapidly-growing Massachusetts Community.* Boston: Department of Sociology, Boston University; 1974.

CHAPTER 10

Continuing Story: Present Plagues

The *MMWR* has always been an unprepossessing publication. In fact, its full title, *Morbidity and Mortality Weekly Report*, is far grander than its appearance. For most of its 50 plus years it has consisted of 4 to 5 sheets of coarse 8- by 10-inch paper stock, printed 2 pages to the side, then folded and stapled on the center crease. Even with some "smartening-up" more recently, it still has no separate cover, no multicolored print or illustrations. It lacks entirely the glossy presentation and prestige of its medical cousins, the *New England Journal of Medicine* and *Journal of the American Medical Association*. But in its humble state, it plays a crucial role. Each week this modest product of the Centers for Disease Control and Prevention (CDC) provides all those people concerned with updates on the nation's current state of health. Much of this information entails ongoing surveillance of infectious diseases, including state-by-state tallies of the "notifiable diseases," that we discussed in Chapter 7. It also affords data from surveys of health risks such as recent smoking patterns or the latest figures on the prevalence of seat belt use. A special feature is the reporting of outbreaks of disease or unusual or unexpected illness such as bursts of diarrhea on cruise ships or clusters of tuberculosis cases occurring in nursing homes.

In the late spring of 1981, the *MMWR* had much that was favorable to report. As the 100th anniversary of Koch's discovery of the tuberculosis bacillus approached, the surveillance tables displayed the progress that had been achieved in mastering infectious disease. The plagues that ravaged the country in its first 2 centuries had all but vanished. Yellow fever was no longer even on the list. Smallpox had not been seen for 30 years and just 2 years earlier had been declared eradicated from the world. Malaria had disappeared as an indigenous disease and now cases appearing on surveillance lists came in from other countries. Polio, which just a quarter of a century before had terrorized the nation, was relegated to the list of "notifiable diseases of low frequency." Just 6 cases of polio would be found in all of 1981, and these were importations or results of vaccine virus. Even tuberculosis, though still reported in some numbers, was declining every year. It claimed only a fraction of the lives it took a century before, when Edward Trudeau moved to the Adirondacks.

It was a euphoric time for public health. So many of the great infectious killers had been "brought to heel." It seemed only a question of time until infectious afflictions would become just memories, relevant primarily to historians. Plans were in place to rid the entire Western Hemisphere of polio, and thoughts of vanquishing tuberculosis from the country were seriously discussed. The capabilities of medical science and public health seemed poised for any challenge. Dozens of potent antibiotics were at the ready for fighting bacterial diseases, new antiviral agents were promising remedy for previously untreatable infections, and robust technology was designing new immunizing agents to short-cut infections before they began.

True, there were still occasional perturbations, as when, in the summer of the country's bicentennial, members of a group attending a convention in Philadelphia fell ill with a new type of pneumonia. But disturbing as that outbreak had been, it was also seen as reassuring for the rapidity with which investigators from CDC responded. It took just months to sort the problem and not only uncover the offending bacterium but describe its mode of spread and suggest the antibiotics needed to effect control. The story of Legionnaire's disease only added to the national self-confidence. Even new diseases were well within our power to control. It was a time of satisfaction, a moment to reflect with pride upon a century of dazzling success. But the moment was about to end.

The cloak of self-deception began to unravel innocuously enough. The June 5 issue of *MMWR* reported 5 cases of pneumonia in young, male patients seen at 3 Los Angeles hospitals over a period of 8 months (1). This scarcely seemed important medical news, let alone an outbreak of any sort. Los Angeles is a huge metropolis and pneumonia a common medical problem. The agent isolated from the patients wasn't even new. It is a rather common parasite carried as a harmless passenger in respiratory tracts of many individuals. The condition carried the tongue-twisting designation *Pneumocystis carinii* pneumonia, or PCP. The 5 young men had all been in good health.

And that was the feature that made staff at CDC take notice. Reports of illness caused by this microbe came almost invariably from patients whose immune systems were severely compromised: those with inborn immune deficiencies, or depletion following aggressive cancer chemotherapy, or deliberate immune suppression following heart or kidney transplantation. These 5 cases were exceptions to that rule. These 5 young men, from 29 to 36, were living full lives when suddenly their health collapsed. Two of the men had died. All had experienced months of fever, and all suffered distressing oral yeast infections, known as thrush, before the pneumonia struck. In addition, all had been infected with another microorganism called cytomegalovirus (CMV), which is common in the environment but rarely causes disease. The cases were peculiar and distressing. So far as the reporting doctors knew, the illnesses were not related. The men did not know one another nor have acquaintances in common. The only similarities appeared to be that all had active, homosexual lifestyles and used inhalant drugs. Still, these were only 5 cases and the report was not even on the front page of the *MMWR*.

Only 1 month later the publication reported on another set of cases (2). This time the disease was an unusual malignancy. It was called Kaposi's sarcoma (KS), and the cases came from New York City as well as California. Again the patients, 26 in all, were younger men, aged 26 to 51. This was a marked departure from the cancer's usual pattern. It was almost always seen in men in their 7th decade or beyond. KS was rare. Its incidence in the United States was thought to be about 2 to 6 cases per 10 million each year. Nor was it an aggressive cancer. Typically, the elderly men who came down with the small purple lesions on their lower limbs had died of something else before the KS had spread. The known exception to this pattern had been in renal transplant patients and others who received immunosuppressive therapy.

The occurrence of 26 cases of KS was decidedly unusual. The cancer registry of New York University had received no reports of the tumor in men under 50 in the previous 10 years, and only 3 cases from this age group had been seen at the University Hospital in the prior 20 (2). The malignancy's behavior was also atypical. It spread aggressively, from the skin to internal organs. By the time the *MMWR* was issued, 8 of the 26 had died. Nor was KS the only problem. Seven of the men had serious infections: yeast, recurrent herpes, and PC pneumonia. All of those tested had also been infected with cytomegalovirus. Again, the only common features seemed to be decimated immune systems and homosexual lifestyle.

By winter it was clear that these case clusters were not isolated episodes. Reports of unusual illnesses were growing. CDC had raised its surveillance antennae and was learning of more and more cases. In just 6 months, episodes of PCP and KS as well as other unusual or "opportunistic" infections* had grown to total 159 (3). Seventy-three of these were KS and 61 PCP; 15 patients had both conditions; and 10 had other infections, including widespread herpes and nervous system infections with a common parasite of cats called *Toxoplasma*. The accompanying illnesses were severe. Patients were racked with persistent fevers and debilitating fatigue. They complained of swollen lymph glands and dramatic loss in weight. Unrelenting diarrhea was common. Thirty-eight percent had died. All but one of these 159 cases was male, their average age was 35, and they lived in 15 states and Washington, DC. Ninety-two percent of those reporting sexual preference stated they were "gay" (homosexual) or bisexual.

No one knew just what was happening. Something appeared to be attacking the immune systems of these men, rendering them susceptible to the bizarre afflictions. It wasn't clear if this was a single disease or many, or what the boundaries were. What was the

---

* An opportunistic infection (OI) is one caused by an organism that only causes disease when host defenses are compromised.

extent of this new plague? How many different guises might it take? How many people were susceptible? And, what was its cause and how was it spread?

Along the corridors of 1600 Clifton Road in Atlanta, Georgia, the home of CDC, these questions were in continuous debate. Soon after the first case reports, a task force had been formed to investigate the new phenomenon, and officers of the Epidemic Intelligence Service (EIS) dispatched to cities like New York, Los Angeles, and San Francisco, where three-quarters of the cases were occurring. As reports accumulated, themes were emerging that provided some direction: the underlying immune deficiency, the multiple unusual infectious agents, and the shared lifestyle. Names were suggested. Self-deprecating gay newspapers were dubbing the problem "gay pneumonia" and "the gay plague." At the CDC, the condition became known simply by its dominant medical feature: acquired immune deficiency syndrome, or AIDS.

"Syndrome," however, is an unsatisfying designation. The term denotes a poorly specified conglomerate of signs and symptoms, lacking in coherence or clear cause. Some working definition was required, even if the dimensions of the problem were unknown. Just as Caverly had struggled to understand the spectrum that comprised polio, epidemiologists at CDC needed to identify the breadth and nuance of this new condition. They needed a definition that would encompass varying stages and severities. In epidemiologic terms, the definition needed to be *sensitive* so that less typical or milder cases, such as Caverly's "aborted polio," would not be missed. There must, however, also be some selectivity. Too broad a net pulls in noncases and gives misleading information—the kind of misclassification we have seen before. Good definitions are also *specific*, meaning that noncases are excluded.

A more recent outbreak of another syndrome offers an example. In March 2003, CDC became aware of a new type of pneumonia, designated SARS, for "severe acute respiratory syndrome" (4). Little was appreciated of the spectrum of the disease, its extent of spread, or cause. All that was known was that the new illness appeared to originate in the Guangdong province of China, had a case-fatality rate of more than 10%, and was spreading. Before data could effectively be gathered to characterize this new threat, some working definition of the problem was required.

The first attempt was basic in the extreme. There were 3 requirements that, if fulfilled, constituted a case of SARS: (1) a temperature
of greater than 100.4°F (38.0°C); (2) a respiratory symptom such as
cough, shortness of breath, or difficulty breathing; and (3) close contact within 10 days of onset of illness with another suspected case or
recent traveler to an area with SARS (4). That's a big net. It meant that
anyone coming from Hong Kong, Hanoi, or Singapore who had a
mild fever and a cold or flu had SARS; quite a few people. CDC was
well aware that the definition lacked specificity. Yet in the early stage
of the outbreak they had to lean toward sensitivity, toward not missing potential cases. As more was learned about the illness, the definition could be refined.

By April 2003 a virus had been identified that seemed responsible for SARS. It was a coronavirus, a member of a family that produces common colds. Once the virus was secured, a test that detected
antibody to the infecting agent was soon in hand. At that point,
laboratory confirmation was possible and could be incorporated
into a more specific definition. Thus, from mid-June to mid-July
2003 the *cumulative* cases of SARS in the United States *fell* suddenly
by 50%, from 418 to 211 (4). The change reflected nothing more than
the chance to test suspected cases for the antibody. When half failed
to show evidence of SARS coronavirus infection, they ceased to
become cases. Specificity had been improved.

The initial definition of AIDS was also broad but principally
because the scope of the syndrome was so difficult to grasp. In the
first iteration it included any patients with Kaposi's sarcoma who
were under 60 years of age, or any patients who had life-threatening
illnesses from so-called opportunistic infections (OIs), like *Pneumocystis*, where there was no underlying illness or reason for immune
deficiency.* The CDC task force suspected that even this definition
was not of sufficient breadth to capture the enlarging plague. "If
immunosuppression is the underlying cause of these conditions,"
the members wrote, "then Kaposi's sarcoma and *P carinii* pneumonia
may represent the 'tip of the iceberg'" (3). How right they were.

---

* Life-threatening illnesses included pneumonia, meningitis, and encephalitis (inflammation of the
    brain). The opportunistic organisms include a cumbersome array of fungi, parasites, bacteria,
    and viruses such as *Cryptococcus, Candida, Toxoplasma, Mycobacteria, Cytomegalovirus*,
    and *Herpes*.

The heads of the hydra were to increase, the list of risk groups grow, and the numbers of cases explode.

As 1982 began, 7 months had elapsed since the first reports appeared, and the cause of AIDS was still a mystery. But several hypotheses by this time were extant. Although initial reports linked the syndrome exclusively to male homosexuals, it soon appeared that intravenous drug users were also involved. A link to some substance used by both groups seemed logical. Many of the gay victims interviewed reported using inhalants containing nitrite chemicals known as "poppers" as sexual stimulants. These as well as other drugs could depress immune response in animals and seemed prime suspects. Others felt the pattern of disease fit that of an infectious agent, one spread by sexual contact. Several leaders of CDC AIDS task force were from the agency's Sexually Transmitted Diseases (STD) Branch and had noted that highly sexually active homosexuals had previously been prone to a variety of STDs such as syphilis, gonorrhea, and hepatitis. It had also been observed that one of the organisms with which AIDS patients had been infected, the cytomegalovirus, could cause depressed immunity, as could a pharmacologic agent used against an amoebic parasite that commonly infected gay men.

The task force had begun an epidemiologic study to help solve the riddle. Hopes were high that good case-control research could cast light upon the cause of AIDS. As the CDC project was moving forward, a group from New York preempted with a case-control report comparing 20 male KS patients with 40 age-matched, homosexual controls (6). A battery of questions ranging from ancestry to "recreational" drug use to sexual behaviors was directed at the 2 groups to search out factors that distinguished those who got KS. Of special interest was exposure to the antiparasitic compound, metronidazole, which was a carcinogen in some animals as well as an immune suppressant. Sexual exposures that might spread an infectious agent, and use of nitrite inhalants were also scrutinized.

The results offered some help. No difference appeared in the use of the antiparasitic drug; that cause could be scratched from the list. But nitrite inhalants and a sexually transmitted agent both gained strong support. When risk ratios were calculated (controlling, of course, for other potentially confusing or confounding factors), both use of amyl nitrite and number of sex partners emerged as strong predictors for KS. AIDS patients were 12 times more likely than controls to have nitrite exposure and twice as likely to have more than 10 sex partners in a month. It was a start to sorting the competing hypotheses, but it still left 2 major possibilities.

Results of the CDC's case-control study added some clarity (7). It included 50 patients with KS and *Pneumocystis* pneumonia and 120 age-matched, gay male controls. As in the New York study, a crucial challenge lay in the choice of controls. It was apparent that, whichever factor was associated with contracting AIDS, it was linked to the homosexual lifestyle. That meant that selecting controls known to be gay risked overmatching. There might be lifestyle factors critical to the development of AIDS that would be masked when both cases and controls were gay. On the other hand, choosing heterosexual controls would likely yield so many differences that little insight would be gained. Many of the variables of interest—prior sexually transmitted diseases, drug use, exposure to medications, and sexual practices—were highly correlated with one another. Teasing out which factors were causally related and which were traveling the coattails was not straightforward.

After statistical techniques had sorted the mélange of risks, the plan proved justified. Despite the concern of overmatching, important differences appeared. Principal among these was the number of male sex partners. Cases averaged 61 per year, more than twice the number of controls. Of equal interest was the finding that the use of nitrite inhalants was similar in the 2 groups. The CDC report confirmed one finding of the earlier study, but not the other. The data supported those who believed AIDS was infectious. But whether infection was due to some familiar organism such as cytomegalovirus, some combination of multiple sexually transmitted agents, or the depredations of a new microbe remained unsolved.

While debates continued on the syndrome's cause, the epidemic continued to reveal itself in new and dreadful ways. In May 1982, the *MMWR* made note of 57 cases of persistent, generalized lymph node enlargement, again in a group of homosexual men (8). Accompanying the swollen nodes were symptoms of fatigue as well as fevers, night sweats, and weight loss. Although these patients did not display life-threatening cancers or infections, the symptoms caused concern. Swollen lymph glands are not unusual. They frequently appear in the neck during sore throat or, more generally, with serious systemic disease. But in these men there was no evidence of infection. Several had their immune systems checked. Their T-helper lymphocytes, cells that are pivotal in recognizing infectious invaders and programming the body's defensive response, were low. It had the same pattern of depleted cellular immunity that was the defining feature of the patients with KS and PCP. It appeared to be a "pre-AIDS" condition. The iceberg was emerging.

One year from the initial report, CDC had uncovered 355 cases of KS; serious opportunistic infections, including PCP; or both (9). These came from 20 states, though California, Florida, New Jersey, New York, and Texas accounted for more than 85%. And 96% of cases were in men, of whom 82% reported having sex with other men. Most women and heterosexual males admitted use of intravenous drugs. Case-fatality rates were high; more than two thirds of the first PCP cases were dead.

Over the next 3 months there was more bad news. In July, 3 cases of PCP were noted in hemophiliacs, victims of a bleeding disorder who require multiple infusions of a clotting factor derived from blood (10). The men were heterosexuals who denied that they used drugs. All had evidence of compromised immunity. In the same month, the *MMWR* also revealed that 34 Haitian immigrants in the United States had been treated for KS and OIs (11). The list of invading adversaries was familiar: *Pneumocystis, Cryptococcus, Toxoplasma, CMV*, and yeast. Among all who were tested, severe immune dysfunction was evident. Most of the new cases were 20- to 40-year-old males, but none admitted sexual contact with other men and only one offered a history of intravenous (IV) drug use.

By December, the *MMWR* told of the deaths of all 3 hemophiliacs and added 4 new cases to this growing group. In the same week, another single case report compounded growing fears. A 20-month-old infant from the San Francisco area was found with multiple infections and decreased T-cell function (12). Because of problems experienced soon after birth, the baby had received transfusions of blood products from 19 different donors. One donor, a 48-year-old male resident of San Francisco, had been in good health when he volunteered his blood in March 1981. Ten months later, he was hospitalized for fever, shortness of breath, and PCP. The evidence was alarming; it suggested a contaminated blood supply.

To cap what was already a disastrous year, the next week brought 4 more case reports of children (13). These infants, however, had received no blood. Two had Haitian mothers and 2 were born to mothers with a history of IV drug use. Three of the 4 children were dead of PCP, as was one of the mothers. More childhood cases, *MMWR* warned, were under investigation.

That made 3 new risk groups for the year: recipients of blood products, infants of mothers with AIDS, and heterosexual, non-drug-using Haitians. Two things were obvious: The epidemic was expanding well beyond the populations first identified, and some infectious agent must be responsible. But the identity of the antagonist remained unknown.

It was not until July 1984 that *MMWR* had major breakthroughs to report (14). But then the news was large, indeed. Three articles in the prestigious journal *Science* described the isolation of a virus that appeared to be the cause of AIDS. In the first instance, researchers in France had cultured a virus from a gay man with generalized lymphadenopathy, the apparent precurser to full-fledged AIDS. Then a similar virus was found among 26 of 72 patients with AIDS by investigators at the U.S. National Institutes of Health. Finally, a researcher in California identified what looked like the same agent in both members of a blood donor-recipient pair who had each developed AIDS.

These revelations were soon the stuff of heated debate. Were these isolates the same virus? Was it in fact the cause of AIDS? Many at CDC and elsewhere were of this mind, but consensus was held hostage for a time while French and American researchers bickered over who should have the credit for the find and what the virus should be called. Each group characterized the virus somewhat differently and supplied it their own name. Declining to take part in the imbroglio, the *MMWR* simply recorded 5 reasons why the isolates were "likely to be the same virus"(14). Although the squabble for discovery primacy continued for some months, the CDC was eager to move on. Settling on a designation proposed by neither rival, they called the new agent *human immunodeficiency virus*, or *HIV*.

And what a virus it turned out to be! Never had our species encountered an organism of such devious design. Like others of the

ilk, its structure is deceptively simple, strands of the genetic substance RNA surrounded in a protein capsule and covered in a fatty
envelope with spikes of sugar-covered protein sticking through (see
Figure 10-1). Like all viruses, it is a parasite, dependent on a living
cell for its support and reproduction. Initially, HIV's operating mode
is typical; it attaches to the host cell wall, then forces its genetic bands
inside. But then, where most viruses settle to the business of usurp-
ing cell machinery to make proteins on their own behalf to build new
viruses, HIV embarks on a different path. The virus brings with it a
special enzyme (protein) known as reverse transcriptase. This
enzyme enables the viral RNA (which usually only directs protein
synthesis) to create DNA, the master genetic material (reversing the
usual process in which DNA produces RNA). This new DNA, containing "programs" necessary to make new viruses, is then incorporated into the host cell's nucleus, into its genetic code. Once there, the

FIGURE 10-1

Human Immunodeficiency Virus Budding from Lymphocyte

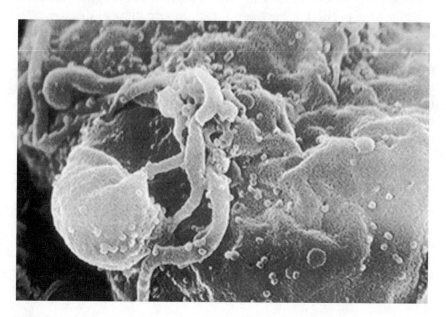

Source: Centers for Disease Control and Prevention.

HIV becomes "invisible;" it cannot be detected by the host's defenses. In this regard, it has gone "underground." Once there, it can remain inactive for months or years but is capable of later activation.

In its choice of cellular host, the human immunodeficiency virus is particularly cruel. The cells it chooses for its home, which ultimately it will destroy, are cells of the immune system. The very cells designed to guard the body from foreign invaders become the refuge and victims of HIV. In particular it is the T-lymphocytes, known as *immune helper cells*, or *CD4 cells*, that fall prey to HIV.*

HIV belongs to a family of viruses designated *Retroviridae* because of their characteristic production of reverse transcriptase. Though retroviruses were discovered almost 100 years ago as a cause of chicken tumors, their role in human illness was not evident until the 1970s. Then the American disputant in the HIV discovery claim found a retrovirus was responsible for unusual cancers (leukemia and lymphoma) in Japan. These tumor retroviruses, called HTLV (for *human T-cell leukemia virus*), differ from the AIDS-producing strains sufficiently to warrant their own designation. HIV belongs to the lentivirus group, named in recognition of the lengthy time occurring between infection and clinical disease.

Several features of the virus make it a formidable foe. Its ability to marry its genetic code with that of the host genome and hide undiscovered has been mentioned. Like others of its RNA brethren, it also shows a tendency to change. In the process of reproduction, in copying genetic code, mistakes are made. Viral offspring can differ from their parents. While these errors, or mutations, are often of no consequence, they sometimes bring advantages to a new virus generation. It is the process of natural selection, which occurs quite slowly in higher life forms. In the fast-replicating world of HIV, however, the changing virus poses a stiff challenge to the host's immune system. New variants can form rapidly enough to stay ahead of immune pursuit. The changing virus presents a constantly moving target.

Another outcome of HIV identification was the rapid discovery of antibodies to the virus in human serum. These could be detected

---

* Several other cells are vulnerable to HIV attack, including another class of immune cells known as *monocytes* or *macrophages*.

several months after infection. It was, of course, an irony that anti-bodies, although in evidence, were not sufficient to eliminate the virus. They did, however, offer a new tool to study AIDS. It now was possible to find infected individuals. While numbers of those ill with "full-blown AIDS" or "pre-AIDS conditions" were generally known, the reservoir of those infected but not yet ill was not. How many of these were there? How likely were they to come down with AIDS? How long would they remain without disease? What was the incubation time from infection to disease? The virus itself was cumbersome to culture and not within the capabilities of most medical laboratories. But several types of antibody tests were soon in hand, and they offered promise of new data by means of *serology* (study of the serum in which antibodies reside).

It would now be possible to estimate the extent of infection across the country and gain insights on the likely incubation peri-od of AIDS. With sequential *serosurveys* one could chart the course of HIV infection, determine the risk in various groups, and track trends of infection over time. Early serosurveys confirmed what many had suspected: Infection varied widely among different seg-ments of the population. Prevalence was alarming in some high-risk groups. Table 10-1 displays results of several surveys gathered by CDC. The range is extreme. Almost half of homosexual and bisexual men in San Francisco are positive, compared with only 2 in 10,000 Red Cross blood donors (15).

TABLE 10-1

Seroprevalence of Human Immunodeficiency Virus in Selected Populations

Population	Positives/1000
Homosexual/bisexual men in San Francisco	490
Intravenous drug users in San Francisco	100
Nevada prison inmates	18
Massachusetts newborns	2.0
U.S. military recruits	1.5
Red cross blood donors	0.2

Source: Based on Centers for Disease Control (15).

One portion of the population about which little was known was the 13 million young adults enrolled in the nation's colleges and universities. This group, "often characterized by a newfound sense of independence, experimentation with sex and sometimes drugs, and a feeling of invincibility" seemed at high risk for HIV (16). But how could data reasonably be acquired on these students? Could one initiate a study in colleges without causing great alarm? Who would volunteer to provide blood samples? How would confidentiality be assured? CDC came up with an ingenious plan. In collaboration with the American College Health Association, they enrolled 19 university health centers to provide samples of serum obtained from students during the routine course of care. The specimen might be taken for a variety of reasons, from a checkup for anemia to assessing high cholesterol. To maintain anonymity, no names were included with the specimens, only age, sex, race, and ethnic group. The 19 chosen institutions were from across the country. That gave good geographic spread. Seventeen selected were public universities since "their student bodies were more likely to be representative of the geographic area in which they were located" (16).

During an 11-month period, almost 17,000 samples of blood were sent to CDC for testing, a sample large enough to give perspective on the magnitude of the problem. The findings were provocative. Thirty specimens were positive; HIV was indeed infecting students. Although the prevalence was not large (two tenths of a percent, when extrapolated to the total population of 13 million), it caused alarm; that was 26,000 infections nationwide. Newspaper wire services picked up the story. They announced that 1 in every 500 college students across the land had HIV.

But extrapolation is tricky business. And this serosurvey, however well intentioned, was not designed to withstand such use. True, the number of samples was large and the campuses selected offered geographic spread. But size and location don't guarantee a representative sample. Before the survey prevalence can be multiplied by 13 million, there must be confidence that the 17,000 students surveyed represent the larger population. This, it seems, is most unlikely. The sample was not a random one, where every student had an equal chance of being included. Only visitors to the health center who had blood specimens obtained are represented. These are a selected set, not only because they seek medical care, but also because they require a blood test. They become a special group, not typical of most of their peers, many of whom never visit the health center let alone have blood obtained. One important reason students have a blood test taken is for suspicion of sexually transmitted disease. It's no surprise that there are instances of HIV infection among the health center patrons. But they are far from typical of the entire 13 million college students in the land.

As soon as the test for HIV became available, concerns arose. How would testing be used? Who would be tested? Who would have access to results? Worries over confidentiality surfaced immediately. Test results are able to reveal not only infection status but lifestyle choices. Fear was widespread that testing would invite discrimination, particularly against gay people. Many groups made clear that testing would not be tolerated unless it was voluntary and the confidentiality of results was guaranteed. Emotions ran high. The decision to be tested was no minor matter; did one really want to know? A negative result brought great relief, but a positive report was ominous in the extreme. Still, many wanted the information. They welcomed the opening of testing facilities that promised anonymity.

One such group of testing sites was developed by the New York State Health Department. These clinics, began providing test results to clients by mid-1985. In addition to offering individual client information, the program compiled anonymous data on the test results to chart trends in facility use and the frequency of positive results. After several years of operation, they published their results (17). These may be seen in Table 10-2a.

The method is typical for serosurveys. Sequential cross-sectional data present the frequency of a health characteristic, in this case HIV infection, over time. The trend looks encouraging. Not only does Table 10-2a show increasing use of the testing facility during the 6-month intervals from January 1986 to December 1987, but the frequency of HIV infection appears to be falling over the 2 years. That is welcome news.

But prevalence trends are often not as straightforward as they seem. The persons tested for HIV in each interval are different; they

TABLE 10-2*a*

Serologic Testing for Human Immunodeficiency Virus in New York State in 4 Time Periods

	Jan. 1986– Jun. 1986	Jul. 1986– Dec. 1986	Jan. 1987– Jun. 1987	Jul. 1987– Dec. 1987
Number tested	2127	2374	4989	7602
Percent positive	14.5	13.6	5.7	4.2

Source: Based on Grabau and Morse (17).

represent different groups and their risks for HIV may not be the same. The Health Department officials who sponsored the testing program also collected information (anonymously) on those who used the service. Some characteristics of these individuals are seen in Table 10-2*b*. The table shows that accompanying the drop in seropositivity are several other changes. The percentages of testees who are male, who have symptoms suggestive of disease, and who come from high-risk groups of homosexual/bisexual and intravenous drug users have fallen. The declining prevalence of HIV among testees cannot be taken as indicative of dropping rates of

TABLE 10-2*b*

Serologic Testing for Human Immunodeficiency Virus in New York State in 4 Time Periods

	Jan. 1986– Jun. 1986	Jul. 1986– Dec. 1986	Jan. 1987– Jun. 1987	Jul. 1987– Dec. 1987
Number tested	2127	2374	4989	7602
Percent positive	14.5	13.6	5.7	
	Test Subject Characteristics			
% male	72.5	66.4	57.8	56.3
% symptomatic	17.7	16.4	8.0	8.0
% intravenous drug user	15.0	14.9	10.9	10.8
% homosexual/bisexual	42.9	39.7	26.1	24.6

Source: Based on Grabau and Morse (17).

infection at large. It appears rather an artifact of the changing demographics (and a priori risk status) of those who use the testing service.

About this same time another well-intentioned attempt to stem the epidemic tide was taking place. A number of state legislatures, determined to do their part to stop the spread of AIDS, considered laws requiring serologic testing for HIV as a prerequisite to obtaining a marriage license. They believed that "screening" prospective couples for HIV status and offering advice might slow the spread of AIDS. Unsuspecting brides and grooms-to-be would be protected from exposure and infection. Thirty-three states contemplated legislation, but only 3 enacted laws, and one of these went through with the experiment. The experience provides a useful lesson in the nuances of broad-based testing programs.

Screening for disease (or for disease risk) is a common strategy in public health prevention. If risk can be identified before disease begins, adverse consequences can often be avoided. Programs that test for elevated blood pressure or high cholesterol are examples. Recall from Chapter 9 that both conditions raise the risk of coronary heart disease. Because neither factor carries outward signs, the only way to learn of increased risk is to test asymptomatic people with a blood pressure cuff or serum cholesterol determination. When elevated blood pressure or cholesterol is found, treatments can be offered that will reduce the chance of CHD. Identifying and remediating conditions before they create problems is *primary* prevention.

In other situations, we lack the ability to head off disease before it starts, but we can detect difficulties in their early stages. Malignancies such as breast and colon cancer provide examples. Mammograms and colon examinations can find tumors that are just beginning, before they become invasive. With appropriate treatment, disease is arrested before it progresses, and years of life are spared. This is *secondary* prevention; disease has begun, but its damage is minimized. Screening programs for primary and secondary prevention are widespread. An effective screening tool correctly classifies those with a condition (for example, breast cancer or candidates for heart attack) as ill or at risk and those who are without risk as normal. Correct classification is never 100%. But the success of screening depends upon achieving the best accuracy possible. There are several aspects of test performance that are important.

As an example, let's consider bone mineral testing as a means of screening to identify people at risk for fractures from osteoporosis. Osteoporosis is another "silent" condition characterized by fragile bones created by low mineral (calcium) content and weakened structure. Disabling fractures of hip and spine and wrist occur with only minor trauma. The problem is particularly severe in older women. Radiographic testing is available to measure bone mineral density (BMD) and can identify individuals with an increased likelihood of fracture.

To see how well a bone density device identifies people who are prone to fractures, we decide to test it in a community. We gather the BMDs of 500 older female residents, then categorize them as having "low" or "acceptable" bone density. We then follow residents for the next 2 years to see who has a fracture (a typical cohort study design). When the results come in, they are as shown in Table 10-3a. The 2 rows of the table identify those categorized as "low" or "acceptable" bone density (110 and 390). The columns indicate the presence or absence of a fracture (25 and 475).

Twenty-five of the 500 (5%) residents sustain fractures in the 2-year interval. How did the test do in identifying them before the fact? It wasn't perfect. Fifteen of the 25 casualties were classed in the "low" bone mineral category, a 60% correct rating; 380 of the 475 people who were free from fracture were properly placed in the "acceptable" bone density bin; 80% correct. These attributes, of correctly classifying those who go on to fracture as "at risk" (low BMD), and those who do not fracture as "not at risk" (acceptable BMD) are called *sensitivity* and *specificity*, respectively. The 10 women that the test said were "acceptable" but who had fractures and the 95 without fractures who had "low" bone density present a problem. These are classification errors, known as *false negatives* and *false positives*, respectively, and demonstrate limitations of the test. On balance, the BMD test does have merit. Of the 110 people who were classified as low, 15, or 13.6%, sustained fractures. This is called *predictive value* and represents the yield or true cases among those with a positive test. The number is more than twice the 5% rate we would expect in the population without applying test results.

The *sensitivity, specificity*, and *predictive value* of screening test are terms that describe performance. The higher all three values are, the better the test works. However, it is difficult to find tests that

TABLE 10-3

a. Results of Bone Mineral Density (BMD) Testing in Predicting Fractures in 500 Women over 2 Years

	Fracture	No Fracture			
				Sensitivity =	15/25 = 60.0%
Low BMD	15	95	110	Specificity =	380/475 = 80.0%
Acceptable BMD	10	380	390	Prevalence =	25/500 = 5.0%
	25	475	500	Predictive value =	15/110 = 13.6%

b. Test Performed on Women 50 Years of Age and Older

	Fracture	No Fracture			
				Sensitivity =	35 = 60.0%
Low BMD	3	99	102	Specificity =	396/495 = 80.0%
Acceptable BMD	2	396	398	Prevalence =	5/500 = 1.0%
	5	495	500	Predictive value =	3/102 = 2.9%

c. Test Performed on Women 70 Years of Age and Older

	Fracture	No Fracture			
				Sensitivity =	30/50 = 60.0%
Low BMD	30	90	120	Specificity =	360/450 = 80.0%
Acceptable BMD	20	360	380	Prevalence =	50/500 = 10.0%
	50	450	500	Predictive value =	30/120 = 25.0%

excel in all dimensions; trade-offs often must be made. We could, for example, identify a greater proportion of fracture cases by raising the BMD level that constitutes a "low" value. This adjustment is not unreasonable. Some people clearly experienced fractures at levels higher than the cut-point we previously defined as low. Raising the bar slightly would include more fracture cases. Sensitivity would improve. However, the improvement would come at a cost. More people in the no-fracture category would be moved to the revised "low" bin as well. This movement would mean more false positives and a lower specificity. We can't have it both ways.

One strategy for bettering test performance is to use it on a population in which there already is a reasonable likelihood of disease. We can screen groups that are known to be at high risk before we offer them the test. In the case of finding fractures, for example, age is known to be a potent predictor. Applying a BMD test to women who are 70 years of age or more produces a result much different from screening those aged 50 and above, as Tables 10-3b and 10-3c demonstrate. These tables show results of BMD testing on 2 age groups with different baseline risks of fracture. Among the younger group, the 2-year risk is low, only 1% of people will have fractures. Because of this low prevalence, the yield from a positive BMD test is also low; only 2.9% of positive tests will occur in someone who goes on to fracture. This means many more false positives (people with a positive test but no fracture) than true positives, and casts doubt on the utility of testing a younger group. For older women, however, testing is more promising. A positive result in this group means a 25% chance of identifying someone who will sustain a fracture in the next 2 years. And that improvement comes without changing the accuracy of the test. It still detects 60% of all fracture cases and correctly classifies 80% of those who don't fracture. The secret lies in selecting subjects for testing who have a higher likelihood of the outcome from the start. In Table 10-3c this prevalence is 10%. So, although there are still false positives, the ratio of true-to-false positives (30/90) is more acceptable at 1 to 3 than occurs with testing of the younger group (3/99) at 1 to 33.

This is where the premarital testing for HIV program got into trouble. The HIV test is exceptionally accurate. Both sensitivity and specificity are well over 90%. On that basis, it seems a perfect tool, ideal for a screening plan to root out HIV. But researchers from Boston knew things are not so simple, that there are hazards in testing a population in which the prevalence of the condition (in this case HIV infection) is very low (18). They calculated the expected outcomes for a program that would initiate premarital testing nationwide. In a single year, that meant about 1.9 million marriages, or 3.8 million testees. Using data from American Red Cross donors, the researchers reckoned that about 35 in every 100,000 people tested would be positive for HIV. They agreed the test was highly accurate and figured on a sensitivity of 98.3% and specificity of 99.8%. Only 2 of every 100 truly infected individuals and 2 in every 1000 noninfected people would be misclassified. Tests don't get much better. Their assumptions produced the numbers in Table 10-4.

The exercise is sobering. For almost 4 million people screened, only 1325 infected people would be found (and a small number, 23, of the infected individuals missed). That number is not encouraging, but is not the worst of the news. Look at the number in the top row of the second column: 7648. Those are the false positives, individuals the test says have HIV infection when they do not. There are 5 of them for every 1 true case. It is an error and a bad one. Consider unsuspecting couples, planning the perfect wedding. Suddenly, they're informed that one is carrying the virus that causes AIDS. Shocking news. Crushing news. News that is completely incorrect. The damage caused by such information can be imagined. Fortunately, large-scale catastrophe could be reduced, as there was a second confirming test that would correctly reclassify most of the false positives. But even then, almost 400 individuals would remain misclassified as HIV infected.

Premarital screening for HIV makes appalling public health policy, particularly considering that even for true positives, the benefits were far from clear. No treatment was available for HIV infection at the time, and national survey data suggested that a substantial proportion of the couples would likely have had sexual intercourse before the tests were done (18). If all this news were not bad enough, the researchers estimated that the cost of such a

TABLE 10-4

Expected Human Immunodeficiency Virus (HIV) Antibody Test Results in a 1-Year National Premarital Screening Program

	HIV Infection	No HIV Infection			
				Sensitivity =	98.3%
Antibody test +	1325	7648	8973	Specificity =	99.8%
Antibody test −	23	3791004	3791027	Prevalence =	0.035%
	1348	3798652	3800000	Predictive value =	14.8%

Source: Based on Cleary et al. (18).

program, including testing and the necessary client counseling, would be in excess of $100 million every year.

Fortunately, most states abandoned plans for premarital testing before the travesty was implemented. Only Illinois embarked upon the program. In the first 6 months of testing, over 70,000 marriage license applicants were screened; 8 were positive (19). That is a prevalence of only 11 in 100,000, one third the estimate the Boston researchers had used in their calculations. (And of those 8, the majority were likely to be *false* positives.) The problem was in screening a population that was low in risk. Nothing in the epidemiology of AIDS suggested that marriage license applicants were an appropriate risk group. Data from the Illinois Public Health Laboratory confirmed that the prevalence of HIV among premarital licensees was only 1/1000 that of high-risk groups within the state (19).

In 1991, the AIDS epidemic was 10 years old. It had been a chastening decade. From the initial cluster of the 5 Los Angeles men, AIDS had grown into a worldwide scourge. U.S. numbers had swelled to 182,000 cases and 116,000 deaths. Not simply an American phenomenon, the disease was now an alarming presence on every continent around the globe. It had progressed far beyond the "gay pneumonia" that was first described; the spectrum of the syndrome now seemed vast. An updated definition from CDC took up 9 pages in *MMWR* (20). This new definition tallied 26 clinical conditions that included 3 malignancies and 14 infectious agents as opportunists to the underlying immune defect.

One addition to the list of clinical conditions was pulmonary tuberculosis. Decades of declining TB rates had been reversed. The lowest rate since case records began in 1953 occurred in 1988: 9.1 new cases per 100,000 population. But in just 3 years the rate had jumped by 14%. A national increase in tuberculosis was disturbing. But was it due entirely to HIV? The epidemiology of the upswing was revealing. When details of the country's cases were examined, the increased rates were found almost exclusively among persons born *outside* the United States. Over an 8-year interval the annual rate of new cases of TB among those who were foreign born had grown from 27.1 to 33.6 per 100,000 population (21). In that same interval, rates for U.S.-born individuals remained virtually unchanged, at 8.1 per 100,000. As immigrants had low prevalence of HIV infection, it seemed that AIDS had little to do with the resurgence in TB.

But such was not the case. A hazard of viewing disease trends with the long lens of a national perspective is loss of detail. In places where both TB and HIV were prevalent, their union, in combination with a faltering pubic health infrastructure, was taking a terrible toll. New York City was the dramatic illustration.

Although historically a city noted for high rates of tuberculosis, New York has also been a model for strong programs aimed at TB control. As far back as the late 19th century, when Health Director Herman Biggs engineered the antispitting regulations noted in Chapter 6, New York City had had aggressive programs to control tuberculosis. Biggs had initiated comprehensive efforts that included active surveillance of cases with visits by public health nurses and isolation of infectious patients (22). But the success brought on by the antibiotic treatment of tuberculosis and the subsequent decline in cases resulted in decreased program funding. Many of New York's treatment facilities were forced to close. The staff of New York's Bureau of Tuberculosis Control, responsible for the largest city in the nation, fell to 140, and the number of TB clinics dropped from 24 to 8. Successful TB therapy requires adherence to a lengthy treatment plan. Close monitoring of patients is essential to success. By 1989, less than half the treatment programs initiated resulted in cures (22). All the reductions had produced predictable results; rates of TB soared. Over 40% had HIV infection.

The course of AIDS was now more clearly understood. Progressing stages in the illness had been delineated. Though not all experience it, for most there is an acute illness at the time of initial infection, as the virus invades and rapidly multiplies. Symptoms are of fever, aching muscles and joints, a rash, and sore throat. But with such symptoms largely indistinguishable from other onslaughts like influenza or infectious mononucleosis, their import is often unrecognized by victims or their doctors. Following this acute phase, an asymptomatic, or quiescent period, sets in.

Far from the 2- to 3-week incubation so characteristic of other infectious agents, the latent phase for HIV appeared to extend for years. New data were producing shocking estimates of 8 to 10 years on average from infection to development of disease; in some cases, even longer. During this interval, there is outward "calm" but turmoil within. The virus and immune system are locked in silent battle. Ultimately, the virus, with its capacity for deception and mutation, prevails. The viral burden in the body grows, the lymph nodes swell, the fever and diarrhea starts, and consuming fatigue sets in*—harbingers of the onslaught of the opportunistic infections and malignancies of "full-blown" AIDS (4). In some ways, this long latency could have been a blessing; patients seemed well and could carry on their usual affairs. But there was also disturbing evidence that they were spreading HIV.

The transmission of the virus of AIDS had also been well characterized. It comes by exchange of body fluids, and that meant risk was wide. Heterosexual as well as homosexual contact spreads the agent as does birth and breastfeeding. Transmission is facilitated by breaches in the body's surface, such as small tears or ulcers of the rectal or vaginal wall or needles penetrating the skin. However, it also became clear that "casual" contact does not transfer HIV. The virus is not passed by coughs or sneezes or even shaking hands. It is not passed on by contaminated clothing or by toilet seats. And, to the great relief of all, the evidence is good that, unlike yellow fever and malaria, AIDS is not spread by insect vectors.

The acquisition of this knowledge was of great help; the patterns of risk had become clear. Along the way, however, some unfortunate confusion occurred. While the epidemiology of AIDS was being revealed, people responded in some unhappy ways. Untoward reactions to disease outbreaks are as old as history. Suspected purveyors of bubonic plague were burned at the stake; citizens fleeing Philadelphia's yellow fever were tarred and feathered. Human nature, unfortunately, has not entirely reformed. Fearing infection, hospital workers refused to deliver meals to rooms of AIDS patients. Others shunned restaurants where waiters were suspected of being gay. Fear inverted the perceived risk from transfused blood; *donations* to the Red Cross fell. Saddest perhaps of all irrational responses was that infected children became pariahs in their schools. It required months of public education and even regulation to correct the damage.

---

* Early symptoms that occur before the opportunistic infections and malignancies may be due to the direct effects of the virus, perhaps from its ability to stimulate production of inflammatory proteins by the host, which in turn damage cells of the nervous, gastrointestinal, and blood-forming systems.

Despite the atmosphere of gloom, several hopeful rays appeared. Substantial progress had been made to improve the safety of the blood supply. In this instance, antibody screening proved an unequivocal success. Testing for HIV made it possible to find contaminated blood and discard infected units. In 1984, more than 700 cases of AIDS were traced to donated blood. In the 6 years following the implementation of required serologic testing in 1985, CDC said fewer than 20 cases annually could be traced to transfusions (23).

Progress was also evident on the antimicrobial front. Medications usually employed to treat established infections with agents like *Pneumocystis* were now being given to immune-suppressed patients *before* they became ill. This preventive or prophylactic use of antibiotics greatly reduced the numbers of individuals who fell ill with PCP. There was also progress on producing counterattacks to HIV itself.

Viruses have long frustrated our antimicrobial efforts. Their uncomplicated structures and symbiotic relationship with human cells offer few chances to interfere with their existence without endangering the host. HIV does offer several such opportunities, however. The special process in which viral RNA is reverse transcribed to DNA is one. A compound known as zidovudine, or AZT, fools the viral enzyme into placing it instead of a critical nucleic acid into the DNA molecule. This substitution creates a faulty molecule that is unable to complete its mission of incorporation into the host genome, and replication of the virus stops. In its first randomized trial in patients, the drug produced such dramatic benefits that the experiment was stopped months before scheduled completion. The drug has downsides, however. Unpleasant side effects develop and hamper continued administration. More ominously, HIV grows tolerant to AZT's suppressing effects.

Drug resistance is another hallmark of a mutating virus. The rapid changes in viral identity that help it escape immune destruction assist its defeat of drugs as well. The enormous variation in viral progeny means that some are likely to have constitutions less susceptible to antiviral medications. These strains particularly prosper when drugs are inadequately administered and blood levels become low. It is an irony that much of HIV's success is due to its propensity to make mistakes. The high transcription error rate is responsible for the many mutations. This feature coupled with the rapid rate of replication and extended length of time within the host make development of drug resistance almost a certainty.

Mutation gives viruses several selective advantages. Their antigenic garb alters to avoid immune detection and transformed genes provide escape from antiviral medications. Another advantage comes with the capacity of some to prey on different animal hosts. Most viruses are fussy. They naturally infect and replicate only in selected cells of a particular animal species. The smallpox virus troubles only humans, as does poliomyelitis. When viruses can prosper in more than one type of host, it is to their benefit. That becomes bad news for humans, however. Viruses that cross the species line threaten us with unfamiliar challenges. Such appears to be the case with HIV. Retroviruses found in chimpanzees and certain species of African monkeys show genetic similarities to HIV strains that cause disease in humans.*

A clearly successful interspecies plague is influenza. The virus responsible for recurrent respiratory epidemics also belongs to the RNA family.** It is another virus that can "change its spots." Key antigens on the influenza virus surface mutate frequently, and the variations that are produced differ sufficiently from one another to escape recognition by the host. Antibodies that are "standing ready" from prior encounters with the virus (either from episodes of illness or immunization with flu vaccine) are of no use. Usually the antigenic changes are relatively small (known as antigenic *drift*), and the new strain of virus results in outbreaks that are limited in scale.

From time to time, however, major antigenic *shifts* produce an influenza virus that is unfamiliar to most of the world, and global outbreaks, or pandemics, occur. These new antigenic strains may come from other species. Influenza viruses are found in horses,

---

* Two types of retrovirus cause human disease in Africa. HIV-1 is responsible for the pandemic and most of the illness in Sub-Saharan Africa. HIV-2 appears to cause less severe disease and is found predominantly in West Africa.
** While many speak of "flu" when referring to a host of mild respiratory and gastrointestinal illnesses caused by a variety of agents, *influenza* belongs to a specific virus family and causes respiratory disease that can be severe.

pigs, and a variety of birds. The virus responsible for the influenza pandemic of 1918, an illness responsible for an estimated 20 to 40 million lost lives, had the antigenic profile of a virus found in swine. When this strain reappeared during the winter of 1976 on a U.S. Army base in New Jersey, it caused considerable alarm. The specter of a repeat pandemic of "swine influenza" was sobering in the extreme. Frantic (and controversial) preparations for this antic-ipated plague included an ill-fated effort plan to immunize the entire U.S. population against swine flu.

For reasons that remain unclear, the pandemic of 1976 never materialized. However, the threat of new viral adversaries emerging from animal strains continues. The coronavirus responsible for SARS shows similarities to viral isolates obtained from masked palm civets, cats that are sold in live animal markets in the Chinese province where the epidemic arose. Transfer of this animal coronavirus has been sug-gested as the origin of the human SARS outbreak. Influenza strains that cause respiratory disease in Southeast Asian fowl are another con-cern. Humans in close contact with infected chickens can "catch" the disease, with serious, sometimes fatal consequences.

Crucial to determining the risk created by cross-species trans-fers is the capacity of the new hosts (humans) to spread disease to one another. In the case of SARS, respiratory transmission seems limited to close contacts. Household members and hospital per-sonnel comprised most of those affected in the outbreak of 2003. Understanding the epidemiology of SARS, its mode of transmis-sion, was critical to containment. Close surveillance that enabled those infected to be promptly identified and isolated during their contagious period proved vital to reducing spread.

After 2 decades of AIDS, the statistics remain grim. The first 20 years of the epidemic saw more than 860,000 cases and 467,000 deaths in the United States alone. At the end of 2002 there were an estimated 360,000 Americans "living with HIV infection or AIDS" (25). On a global scale, the news was worse. An estimated 40 million people had HIV/AIDS (see Figure 10-2). Five million new infections were occurring annually, as were 3 million deaths (25). Most affected is Sub-Saharan Africa, where 25 to 28 million people are believed to be infected. In Africa, transmission of the virus has a different pattern from the epidemic in North America and Western Europe.

FIGURE 10-2

Adults and Children Estimated to be Living with HIV/AIDS as of End 2003

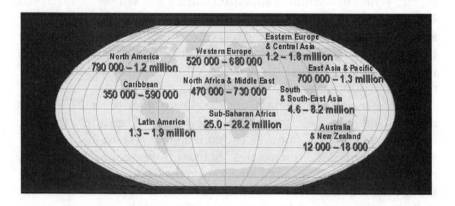

Source: World Health Organization (World Health Organization. AIDS epidemic update: December, 2003. Website, http://www.who.int/hiv/pub/epidemiology/epi2003/en/).

The spread is almost entirely through heterosexual intercourse; females make up 60% of cases, compared with only 20% in North America. In some African countries, more than 20% of people from 15 to 49 years of age are thought to be HIV positive. The disease has destroyed entire families.

There continues to be some progress in the United States. More drugs have been developed to control the replication of HIV. Three classes of compounds are now available, each acting on a different aspect of viral reproduction. Patients on these new treatments have fared well. Viral presence in the blood drops dramatically and CD4 lymphocyte counts improve. The annual number of AIDS deaths in the United States has fallen from a peak of 50,000 in 1995 to 16,000 in 2002. Many individuals are now free from the ravages of opportunistic infections and can carry on with active lives. However, this success does not mean victory. Antiretroviral medications suppress the virus but do not eliminate it. If therapy is discontinued, the virus reemerges from sequestered nooks and problems begin again. Moreover, the mutating ability of HIV means that drug resistance continues as a problem with these newer agents as well. Chances of avoiding resistant strains increase when patients are given multiple drug treatment with agents that attack the virus at varying points of vulnerability. But multidrug regimens are challenging. Dosing is complicated; there are often many pills to take on empty stomachs at inconvenient intervals. There are unpleasant and sometimes serious side effects as well. The drugs are expensive and the commitment to therapy must be (as far as we know) lifelong. Extraordinary diligence is required, and adherence is often less than complete. It is estimated that fewer than 50% of patients who begin therapy are adequately adherent to the plan 1 year after starting. Poor adherence raises the likelihood of relapse and fosters development of drug-resistant strains.

We've corrected some lapses as well. New cases of tuberculosis are once more in decline. Since the resurgence peak in 1992, rates have come down by 50%. New York City reinvested in the Bureau of TB Control (22). Staffing was quadrupled, and the budget grew from $4 million to $40 million in 7 years. Outreach workers fanned out to visit patients in homes, workplaces, street corners, and park benches to ensure adequate treatment. The proportion of patients completing therapy rose to 90%. Institutions such as homeless shelters, jails, and hospitals increased their efforts at infection control, with gratifying results. In just 2 years the city's cases fell by 21%. It was a matter not of know-how but of will.

The story of AIDS continues to unfold. Since 1981, *MMWR* has published over 400 reports on the evolution of the epidemic. There will be more to come. Our struggle with the disease has been chastening. It certainly cured complacency. AIDS has shown how far we are from mastering biology. A simple particle of only 8 chromosomes can alter cells in ways that we still only partly understand and change before our drugs or defenses can gain control. The epidemic has reminded us how complex control of disease in human beings can be. Its nuances have touched on every aspect of our social selves. We have mapped the means by which the disease is spread, yet we cannot contain it. Behaviors that transmit the virus continue. The latest annual reports suggest new cases of AIDS are rising in the United States. Just how and with what authority we can alter this escape us.

New threats continue to emerge. In the 2 decades since *MMWR* signaled the start of AIDS it has published reports on bovine spongiform encephalopathy (mad cow disease), hantavirus pulmonary syndrome, and West Nile encephalitis as well as SARS. Each one of these attacks was new. What is more, the CDC reminds us that, while rates of smoking have declined, and deaths from CHD have dropped, the weight of Americans has ballooned, diabetes diagnoses grown, and heavy use of alcohol increased—omens that new chronic plagues await.

On the other hand, we have moved ahead. There are lessons we have mastered in the centuries since Mather railed at opponents of inoculation and Rush bled yellow fever victims while his Philadelphia brethren shot muskets in the air to ward off the miasmas. We've found out some things about ourselves and about what makes us sick. We've discovered we are far more than a collection of humors that fall in and out of equilibrium. Symptoms of illness are not simply reactions to crude shifts in blood or bile but responses of preprogrammed cells with highly detailed purposes. Nor are we helpless pawns before a malign environment. The longstanding fears of disease-inducing vapors that saturate the air are put to rest. Decaying waste and stagnant swamps are not themselves the causes of poor health. We have uncovered more complex relationships between illness and the surrounding world. The microorganisms most proximately linked with sickness may breed in waste or rely on insect intermediaries that reproduce in stagnant pools. Toxic vapors may not come from organic soils but from the smoke of burning leaves that we intentionally inhale. As knowledge of the links between ourselves as hosts, inducing agents, and the environment has grown, we've seen opportunities to break causal chains by taxing cigarettes or reducing mosquito habitat.

Likewise, the perception of the role of human factors in the cause and course of illness has evolved. We've long abandoned the fatalistic view of Zabdiel Boylston's antagonists that illness is brought down on us to punish original sin. Our theories have also progressed from belief that willful moral failings make us sick. While for a while newfound microorganisms seemed sufficient to explain disease, we've come to acknowledge that our behaviors do contribute to our ills. Stressful life events can activate latent tuberculosis and fat-filled diets tax our hearts. Microbes are spread when needles are shared or intercourse is unprotected.

We've found that theories of illness are barren without supporting evidence. Carefully collected facts both to support and challenge our hypotheses are critical to furthering our knowledge of cause. Anecdotes and opinion, no matter how fervently promoted, cannot replace sound evidence. We've learned that data must be gathered with care. Selecting biased samples or misclassifying subjects leads to inaccurate results. To understand how disease occurs we must appreciate its natural variability and course and realize that some relationships are mere coincidence. Only with proper comparisons can the roles of chance and natural course be teased from cause. The same principles apply to seeking cures.

We've developed useful tools to help us study health. Over the years we've learned to diagnose and classify disease with consistency. Research designs are now available to aid our causal searches with structured comparisons. There are now methods to sort the roles of competing explanations and neutralize confounding factors such as age. We've learned to conduct experiments in human groups to test preventatives and therapies. In the process we've found the means to lessen bias by random assignment, double blinding, and use of placebo controls. The list is an impressive one and it goes on.

In hindsight, Cotton Mather set the tone for all this in his low-ceiling-beamed back hall. He counseled young Ben Franklin to make lessons of bumps on the head, to use experience to chart his future path. Collectively, it seems, we've taken that advice. The intervening years have shown us capable of gaining from experience. Our task remains to keep on learning.

REFERENCES

1. CDC. *Pneumocystis* pneumonia—Los Angeles. 1981; 30:250–252.
2. CDC. Kaposi's sarcoma and *Pneumocysitis* pneumonia among homosexual men—New York City and California. *MMWR Morb Mortal Wkly Rep.* 1981; 30:305–307.
3. Epidemiologic aspects of the current outbreak of Kaposi's sarcoma and opportunistic infections. *N Engl J Med.* Jan 28 1982; 306(4):248–252.

4. CDC. Outbreak of severe acute respiratory syndrome—
   worldwide, 2003. *MMWR Morb Mortal Wkly Rep.* 2003;
   52:226–228.

5. CDC. Update: severe acute respiratory syndrome—
   worldwide and United States, 2003. *MMWR Morb Mortal
   Wkly Rep.* 2003; 52:664–665.

6. Marmor M, Friedman-Kien AE, Laubenstein L, et al. Risk
   factors for Kaposi's sarcoma in homosexual men. *Lancet.*
   May 15 1982; 1(8281):1083–1087.

7. Jaffe HW, Choi K, Thomas PA, et al. National case-control study of Kaposi's sarcoma and Pneumocystis carinii
   pneumonia in homosexual men: Part 1. Epidemiologic
   results. *Ann Intern Med.* Aug 1983; 99(2):145–151.

8. CDC. Epidemiologic notes and reports persistent, generalized lymphadenopathy among homosexual males.
   MMWR Morb Mortal Wkly Rep. 1982; 31:249–251.

9. CDC. Epidemiologic notes and reports update on
   Kaposi's sarcoma and opportunistic infections in previ-
   ously healthy persons—United States. *MMWR Morb
   Mortal Wkly Rep.* 1982; 31:300–301.

10. CDC. Opportunistic infections and Kaposi's sarcoma
    among Haitians in the United States. *MMWR Morb
    Mortal Wkly Rep.* 1982; 31:353–354, 360–361.

11. CDC. Epidemiologic notes and reports *Pneumocystis
    carinii* pneumonia among persons with hemophilia
    A. *MMWR Morb Mortal Wkly Rep.* 1982; 31:365–367.

12. CDC. Epidemiologic notes and reports. Possible transfusion-
    associate acquired immune deficiency syndrome
    (AIDS)—California. *MMWR Morb Mortal Wkly Rep.* 1982;
    31:652–654.

13. CDC. Unexplained immunodeficiency and opportunistic
    infections in infants—New York, New Jersey, California.
    MMWR Morb Mortal Wkly Rep. 1982; 31:652–654.

14. CDC. Antibodies to a retrovirus etiologically associated
    with acquired immunodeficiency syndrome (AIDS) in
    populations with increased incidences of the syndrome.
    MMWR Morb Mortal Wkly Rep. 1984; 33:337–339.

15. CDC. Human immunodeficiency virus in the United States: A review of current knowledge. *MMWR Morb Mortal Wkly Rep.* 1987; 36 (suppl S6):22.

16. Gayle HD, Keeling RP, Garcia-Tunon M, et al. Prevalence of the human immunodeficiency virus among university students. *N Engl J Med.* Nov 29 1990; 323(22):1538–1541.

17. Grabau JC, Morse DL. Seropositivity for HIV at alternate sites. *JAMA.* 1988; 260:3128.

18. Cleary PD, Barry MJ, Mayer KH, Brandt AM, Gostin L, Fineberg HV. Compulsory premarital screening for the human immunodeficiency virus. Technical and public health considerations. *JAMA.*1987; 258:1757–1762.

19. Turnock BJ, Kelly CJ. Mandatory premarital testing for human immunodeficiency virus. The Illinois experience. *JAMA.* Jun 16 1989; 261(23):3415–3418.

20. CDC. 1993 revised classification system for HIV infection and expanded surveillance case definition for AIDS among adolescents and adults. *MMWR Morb Mortal Wkly Rep.* 1992; 41:RR–17.

21. McKenna MT, McCray E, Onorato I. The epidemiology of tuberculosis among foreign-born persons in the United States, 1986 to 1993. *N Engl J Med.* Apr 20 1995; 332(16):1071–1076.

22. Frieden TR, Fujiwara PI, Washko RM, Hamburg MA. Tuberculosis in New York City—turning the tide. *N Engl J Med.* Jul 27 1995; 333(4):229–233.

23. Selik R, Ward J, Buehler J. Trends in transfusion-associated acquired immune deficiency syndrome in the United States, 1982–1991. *Transfusion.* 1993; 33:890–893.

24. CDC. *HIV/AIDS Surveillance Report* 2002; 14:1–23.

25. World Health Organization. AIDS epidemic update: December, 2003. Website, http://www.who.int/hiv/pub/epidemiology/epi2003/en/.

INDEX